OXFORD MEDICAL PUBLICATIONS

Essentials of geriatric medicine

Essentials of geriatric medicine

Second edition

GEORGE F. ADAMS, C.B.E., M.D., F.R.C.P.

formerly Honorary Professor of Geriatric Medicine,
Queen's University of Belfast, and Visiting Professor
of Geriatric Medicine, Department of Medicine,
University of Manitoba

OXFORD

OXFORD UNIVERSITY PRESS

NEW YORK   TORONTO

1981

Oxford University Press, Walton Street, Oxford OX2 6DP
London   Glasgow   New York   Toronto
Delhi   Bombay   Calcutta   Madras   Karachi
Kuala Lumpur   Singapore   Hong Kong   Tokyo
Nairobi   Dar es Salaam   Cape Town
Melbourne   Auckland
and associate companies in
Beirut   Berlin   Ibadan   Mexico City

First published 1977
Reprinted 1978
Second edition 1981

British Library Cataloguing in Publication Data

Adams, George F.
  Essentials of geriatric medicine.—2nd ed.
  —(Oxford medical publications)
  1. Geriatrics
  I. Title
  618.97   RC952
  ISBN 0-19-261352-9

Typeset by Latimer Trend & Company Ltd, Plymouth
Printed and bound in Great Britain by
William Clowes (Beccles) Limited, Beccles and London

TO MARY

Preface to the second edition

For this edition new sections have been added on theories of ageing, retirement, domiciliary visiting, and geriatric dermatology. It is not known yet why or how tissues age, but speculation about the process is increasingly being replaced by facts from microbiological research, and it seemed appropriate to include a brief review of their influence on contemporary hypotheses. People are retiring earlier and living longer, so the scope and possibilities of pre-retirement counselling have been discussed. Visits to assess the medical and social problems of elderly invalids in their homes have a unique value in consultant geriatric medical practice. I am grateful to Dr. E. W. Knox for a thoughtful and perceptive essay on this topic, and to Dr. Susan Burge for an account of some skin disorders of old age.

The Table of morphological age changes and their effects on different systems was well received in the original book. It seems to fulfil its purpose in distinguishing effects which may be accepted as 'normal' consequences of ageing from those which should arouse concern as pathological trends. The Table has been revised and recast to include new data. The passages on dementia, falls in old age, endocrinological age changes, and the treatment of parkinsonism and hypothermia have been rewritten, and some minor changes were necessary in other sections.

Social service resources and skills were mentioned in the previous edition as essential to the successful management of precariously dependent old people. In response to some critics these preventive care services have now been discussed in more detail and my thanks are due to Mrs. E. A. Harrison, Senior Medical Social Worker, for this contribution.

I wish to acknowledge my indebtedness and express my thanks to the authors and editors I have quoted, and to reviewers and friends for encouraging and constructive comments, especially to Dr. T. W. Tinsley, Dr. N. F. Moore, Dr. T. J. Ryan, Dr. G. M. Komrower, Professor R. G. Macfarlane, and Commander W. Ackworth for giving their time and consideration to helpful criticism of the new sections, and to Mrs. G. Dixon for her expert secretarial help.

I am most grateful to Mrs. Alison Langton and the Oxford University Press for encouragement to produce a new edition, and for their permission to draw upon papers from the proceedings of the Vichy World Conference on Aging (*Aging: a challenge to science and society*, Vols 1–3) in advance of publication. I am grateful also to MTP Press of Lancaster for permission to reproduce Table 4.

Despite the length necessarily added by revision, I hope the book still provides a concise presentation of essentials primarily for students of medicine, but useful also to anyone concerned with the care of old people.

Oxfordshire
May 1981   G.F.A.

Preface to the first edition

The question 'What is geriatrics?' is often asked but seldom answered well because there is less scientific discipline than philosophy in its practice. In the United Kingdom, which has led in its development, it is defined as 'the branch of general medicine concerned with the clinical, preventive, remedial, and social aspects of illness in the elderly'. This describes the range of positive, constructive, clinical practice available to the geriatric physician in contrast to the popular, but negative, view of his work as no more than a 'clinical undertaker', relieving his colleagues of long-stay and terminal-care problems. However, just as 'the essence of food cannot be expressed in terms of calories' neither can the philosophy of geriatric medicine be expressed by the lifeless words of a definition. It cannot explain the absorbing range of diagnostic and remedial opportunities in medical work with old people. It cannot describe the rewards of involvement in their unexpected recoveries after critical illness, in devising successful management of their protracted disabilities, or in assuring them of comfort and dignity in their last hours. Nor can it reveal the attractions of their personalities as patients; their wisdom, often concealed behind an outward façade of reticence; their humour; their courage in adversity; and their dislike of insincerity or bogus attitudes (especially in professional advisers). The term 'medicated survival' is a misnomer. People who have lived to a ripe old age are usually 'good lives' and owe their longevity less to medical science than to their own genetic endowments combined with the true cornerstones of survival— warmth, food, fluids, and companionship.

Knowledge of geriatric medicine derived only from hospital experience gives a grossly distorted view of old age, because it is biased so much by a heavy mortality and a high rate of continuing care amongst the older patients. They, however, only represent a small fraction of the population of old people. When a count is made of all the over-sixties cared for by institutions of any kind (including hospitals, nursing homes, and sheltered housing), it will be found that not more that six to eight per cent of the total population of old people are in them; the rest are either looking after themselves, or being looked after, in private dwellings of some sort, and the medicine of old age, therefore, should be home- and not hospital-orientated. The family doctor, who provides this domestic medical care, is best able to appreciate the resilience, the grit, and the resolute determination of the vast majority who hold on to their independence as long as they are able.

Most old people ask little of their doctors unless they feel really ill, or their range of activity is narrowing towards significant loss of independence, or they are so handicapped that they need support to maintain ordinary standards of hygiene and self-care. If they have lost the insight to ask for medical advice in

such circumstances, their need for it is genuine indeed. The problem too often is
that the victim waits too long to ask.

This is a third edition, and in the original introduction it was suggested that
'the attractions of geriatric medicine are appreciated late rather than early in a
medical lifetime and it has little appeal as a prospective career to the student or
the new graduate'. Perhaps it would have been wiser to write 'little immediate
appeal'. Whilst few students may consider specializing full-time in geriatrics,
most of them recognize the need for special attention to the problems of ageing.
They appreciate teaching of geriatric medicine as a part of their medical
education, and they enjoy geriatric medical practice in a well-organized department of geriatric medicine as part of their postgraduate training. However,
it is well known that amongst the reasons doctors have had for turning to
geriatrics, dedication to the care of the elderly is not the most prominent; there
is truth, but perhaps too much cynism, in the view of this expressed by Wright
and Simpson (1967) that 'The satisfaction it offers comes, not from being
surrounded by senility and chronic sickness, but from meeting a challenge that
has beaten others, and from being a pioneer.'

The reasons for reservations about a career commitment in geriatrics in early
medical life are easy to understand. The investigation and diagnosis of diseases in
childhood and early adult life are more straightforward, and cure is often more
dramatic, than amelioration and slow partial rehabilitation of the elderly.
Young people in a hurry find their patience is overtaxed by tedious geriatric
history-taking and examination; besides they have difficulty enough at this stage
in recognizing deviation from what is considered normal for the child or healthy
adult. Age changes add another perplexing dimension. Distinguishing those
which can be accepted without concern, from pathological changes which need
investigation, is complicated frequently by mental and physical evidences of
disintegration in the nervous system. Neurology is difficult at the best of times,
and psychiatry even more so. Some students cannot stand working with old-
agers; others do not want to practice clinical medicine at all.

However, even if it must be accepted that few undergraduates will find instant
appeal in geriatric medicine, they must be informed about an essential
minimum—a core content, of its science, its philosophy, and its art. This is
necessary, if only because of the sheer size of the growing problems of an ageing
society. In a lecture to the Royal College of Physicians and Surgeons of Canada
in January 1976, Dr. W. B. Spaulding observed that the ideal core content of a
subject in medical education should be individualized, revised often (to prune
obsolescence), and applicable to clinical problems, because human memory is
fallible and it is essential to have ready access to vital data. This booklet is an
attempt to fulfil these criteria. It is a personal view of core knowledge of geriatric
medicine compiled partly from lecture notes, partly from the references given,
and partly from things heard or read—sources long since forgotten. It is a
foundation of basic data to be administered to students in small, repeated,
infusions of teaching—clinical teaching, not sterile lectures, throughout all their
hospital years; to be extended by visits to the aged at home and in other
accommodation outside hospitals; and to be built on by further reading.

This should include some of the philosophy distilled from long experience by some of the authors given in the list of references, and the splendid essays written by Eckstein, Platt, Sheldon, and Welford deserve special mention. The bibliography has been chosen with care, but is by no means wholly representative.

The main aim of medical education probably should be to ensure that the 'compleat physician' acquires a happy combination of the science and the art of medicine in the service of mankind (Gilchrist 1963). This desire for proper recognition of the uniqueness of the individual, and for balance in medical teaching between science and humanism, is constantly reiterated in medical writing. It may best be fulfilled by complementing the science of general medicine with the art of geriatrics.

Oxfordshire   G.F.A.
February 1977

Acknowledgements

I WISH to acknowledge my indebtedness to Dr. J. A. MacDonell, Head of the Section of Geriatric Medicine, for the suggestion that I should write this handbook, and for the opportunity to do so, made possible by the kind invitation from the Department of Medicine of the University of Manitoba to come to Winnipeg as Visiting Professor in Geriatric Medicine. I am grateful to Dr. J. P. Gemmell, Dr. J. A. Hildes, and Professor Ronald Cape for critical comment and suggestions, to Miss M. C. Day and Mrs. E. M. Newman for secretarial help, and to Mrs. M. Protosavage for her patience and care in preparing the manuscript.

Contents

xiv   *Contents*

1 The process of ageing

Physiological and pathological concepts

Man, like other biological species, appears to have a genetically determined *life span*: a fixed age limit unchanged in recorded history. Modern medicine and social progress since 1900 have greatly extended the average expectation of life at a given age, i.e. *life expectancy* (p. 20). It is thought that at least another ten years could be added to the expectation of life at birth if the main killing diseases (heart disease, stroke, and cancer) were eliminated, but prevention of disease is not expected to alter human life span, only to enable more people to reach its limit and to die in physiological decline on about their one-hundredth birthday (Hayflick 1976). As things are, only exceptional people (Sheldon's 'aristocracy of old age'), survive to be really fit and active in mind and body beyond 75 years of age.

Three phases of mammalian life have been described (Horrabin 1968):

1 *Embryonic life:* dependent on maternal support for the development of the systems necessary to withstand environmental challenge
2 *Healthy adult life:* when the organism remains in equilibrium with the environment by maintaining cell function and repair
3 *Senescence:* as maintenance and repair gradually becomes less effective, and cells die, and organ function declines

There are probably as many definitions of 'age' as there are theories of its cause. The word is used unambiguously only 'when it refers to the passage of time', i.e. chronological age; but in the more general sense of 'the decline of vitality', 'reduced biological efficiency', 'diminished response to environmental challenge', or 'progressive decrement in the ability of the organism to react to stress' (to quote some of the attempts at definition), the ageing process may involve factors other than time, such as mental or physical illness, deprivation in various guises, trauma, or other kinds of stress. These add to or accelerate the impaired function and inexorable decline of normal ageing, and it is usual, therefore, to suppose that age, as it impinges on the development and maintenance of the human organism, is the sum of these two processes: time-related, involutional 'physiological' changes, and wear-and-tear, disease, or stress-induced 'pathological' changes. In practice it is difficult to dissociate one from the other and it is difficult also to devise measurements or estimates of normal age changes whether by the study of physiological capacity, biochemical function, or of morbid anatomy and histopathology. For example, decline in the capacity for physical work is a recognized feature of normal ageing, and an old person will often attribute it simply to muscular weakness, another commonplace in old age. Muscle strength can be tested by an instrument which gives an accurate register of strength of grip, a quality which declines by almost 50 per cent between the ages of 30 and 75. But what, in fact, is being measured?

Any physical performance reflects the combined capacities of various body systems: muscle strength, neuro-muscular co-ordination, cardio-respiratory efficiency in the supply of properly oxygenated blood in appropriate quantities to brain and muscle, waste removal by the kidneys, and the maintenance of a constant metabolic and biochemical *milieu intérieur*. All the systems concerned in these mechanisms will be impaired in some degree by age changes. However, the muscular effort involved in grip makes demands not only on the nervous pathways of sensory input, cortical integration, and motor response but also on intellectual, emotional, and personal factors which determine endurance and the attitudes and responses of individual 'psychomotor performance'. Estimates must take account also of extraneous physical limitations imposed by degenerative changes in aged bones, joints, muscles, and circulation. A feeble grip might represent something quite different from muscular weakness: perhaps reluctance to provoke pain in an arthritic hand, an irresolute attitude, or apathy and lack of incentive attributable to depression. It must be acknowledged, therefore, that differentiation of 'normal' from 'pathological' ageing is often artificial, but it is useful when applied to distinguish preventable, or reversible, disease processes (which may hasten decline in old age) from age changes which are irreversible and have to be accepted, and it helps to simplify consideration of the ageing process to think of it in this way.

Time-changes attributed to ageing

The time-changes attributed to ageing that have attracted most research interest are:

1 the failure of mitosis in tissues composed of cells which divide and regenerate

2 the deterioration of more specialized non-dividing cells (particularly neurons and muscle cells) leading to a loss of functional efficiency and then to disintegration and death

3 the changes in connective-tissue protein which cause increased rigidity and loss of elasticity in the collagens and elastins comprising more than half of the protein in mammalian bodies, binding their skin, muscle, nerves, and much else

It has been shown, *in vitro*, that specific cells such as fibroblasts only divide a certain number of times (Hayflick 1965). Older cells divide less often, limited, apparently, by chromosomal aberrations and mitotic eccentricities which alter capacity for cell growth and multiplication. Non-dividing cells in tissue culture lose cytoplasmic constituents such as their mitochondria, RNA, and intracellular enzymes. As they shrink, the nucleus becomes smaller and lipofuscin (the wear-and-tear pigment) accumulates as yellow granules in the cytoplasm.

Theories of ageing

There has always been more theory than fact offered to explain these phenomena, but research interest in the physiology of senescence is growing and the technology of cell culture, successful in bringing so much progress in virology and immunology, is being turned increasingly on age changes in tissues in search of the data necessary to test various hypotheses and to determine promising new lines of investigation. Details of these, and of theoretical aspects of ageing, are available in symposia edited by Rockstein (1974) and by Danon and Shock (1981), and in a review by Williamson and Johnson (1980). The following outline, condensed from these sources, is a brief account of age changes demonstrated at the cellular level by studies of molecular biology, protein chemistry, and immunological function in tissue cells, and of the effects of ageing on homeostasis and the mechanisms that control performance and maintain the integrity of the whole organism.

Ageing in tissues
Cells of different tissues appear to age in different ways and at different rates. Functional decline in tissues made up of non-dividing cells such as the specialized elements of the nervous system and muscle seems to be determined by the rate of cell loss; whereas ageing is deferred in tissues with mitotic cells, in some, perhaps, by multiplication of stem cells to compensate for those lost by age changes. This does not imply that tissues (or individuals) age and die because their cells lose their capacity to replicate. This is only one of many functional properties of cells that change with time, and ageing is more probably attributable to age-related deterioration in biological function, and in behaviour, of cells that antedates—or simply accompanies—loss of the capacity to

proliferate. Some cells show primary ageing, apparently independently of their immediate environment; in others ageing is secondary to changes in other systems. For example, skin or corneal grafts could far outlive their host, and these tissues appear to age because their owner ages; on the other hand, muscle tissue atrophies secondary to ischaemia, disuse, hormone deficiency (testosterone), or motor nerve lesions.

Age brings to some tissues accumulations of substances that are of no apparent use, such as cholesterol in arteries and the gall bladder, chalk in cartilage, and lipofuscin, prominent in the post-mitotic cells of the nervous system, heart muscle, kidney, adrenal cortex, and gonads. (Lipofuscin is thought to be an incomplete breakdown product of degenerating lysosomes.)

Other cellular changes relating to the tissues of individual body systems follow later in Table 1 (pp. 10–17).

Ageing of the cell at the molecular level
The main functions of DNA are self-replication in mitosis and transcription of messenger RNA contributing to protein synthesis. Damage to DNA leads to inaccurate transcription, failure to produce appropriate proteins, and defective cell division. The appearance of chromosomal aberrations in some ageing cells has encouraged various theories of ageing based on impaired DNA function:

1 DNA replication and RNA transcription require appropriate enzymes at all stages, and the enzymes themselves are the products of precise protein synthesis. *Defective enzymes*, therefore, might in some way be a consequence of age-dependent error—an example given by Hayflick (1974) being the synthetase enzymes involved in the assembly of amino acid chains into proteins on the RNA template. A build-up of errors in enzyme-producing molecules could bring about a burst of 'nonsense' protein or of lethal mis-specified proteins (much as a faulty machine tool would produce faulty parts). This is an imaginative theory in that although errors and nonsense insertions are known to occur, as they are likely to destroy the cell it is difficult to devise reliable tests to establish this as a cause of ageing.
2 *Mutation:* defined as faulty transcription of DNA during mitosis, appears spontaneously with age, or in response to radiation. Genetic changes and altered protein synthesis might be expected as adverse effects from the accumulation of random mutations. A switch in the role of key enzymes, and loss of cell specificity, could then lead to cumulative errors and 'ageing' of cells; the output or the activities of proteins produced for extracellular functions (digestive enzymes, hormones, or neurotransmitters) might be altered or lost; changes in

cell-surface antigens could lead to disordered immune responses and autoimmune disease; or faulty genetic repressor production could cause de-differentiation and atrophy of cells (a common feature of ageing tissues).

3 *Cross-linkage:* the bonds which form the double strands of intra-cellular protein molecules, especially those surrounding the DNA helix, may become 'cross-linked' by the accidental attachment of chemically active, unwanted, migrant molecules which cut short normal replication of DNA causing mutation or cell death. In theory there are always plentiful migrants such as these derived from formal-dehyde and other byproducts of normal metabolic processes. Defence mechanisms normally protect against excessive cross-linkage, but when they fail, conglomerations of cross-linked macromolecules may create amorphous deposits such as hyalin and amyloid or induce other age-dependent deterioration.

4 *Free radicals:* these are highly reactive molecular fragments, a prop-erty they owe to an unpaired electron which enables them to use free energy to attack neighbouring molecules by oxidation. They are be-lieved to promote cross-linkage, causing chromosomal aberrations and other intracellular havoc. (Antioxidants such as Vitamin E inactivate free radicals but it has yet to be proved that they retard ageing or prolong life in humans.)

5 *Extraneous factors:* ischaemia, toxins, disuse, or deprivation are am-ongst possible extracellular origins of impaired metabolism and func-tions within the cell. Adverse effects on *mitochondria* could reduce the output of cell energy; on *ribosomes* cause defective protein synthesis; and on *lysosomes* release an excess of unwanted enzymes to disorganize the cell.

These hypotheses imply that the intracellular damage attributed to the underlying agencies occurs owing to impaired body defences. The immune system and the nuclear and cytoplasmic defence mechanisms developed in early life normally identify aberrant molecules and pro-tect the genetic apparatus, cell constituents, and their functions from such ill-effects by 'repair, catabolism, and extrusion'. With age, or because of it, or as a source of age changes, defences fail, weakened per-haps by a lifetime of exposure to adverse factors of one kind or another. However, none of these, alone, can provide the basis for a theory to account for all aspects of ageing, and direct evidence to support their theoretical effects may never be forthcoming. Amongst possible causes that may bring them into play are *radiation*, already mentioned as a source of aberrant cells, *viruses*, known to alter genes and effect neo-plastic change in certain circumstances, and *autoimmune phenomena*.

6   *The process of ageing*

Immunity and ageing

Age changes in the immune system, decreased immune reactivity to foreign antigens, and increased autoimmune reactions in senescence have been credited with a primary pathogenetic role in the process of ageing in man. Lymphocytes which differentiate within the thymus or under its endocrine control (T-cells) mediate cellular immune functions and, by the secretion of specific mediators called lymphokines, control the function of macrophages and the production of specific antibody by B-lymphocytes. These cells interact to create a balanced state of immunological surveillance in health.

With ageing, reactivity of both T- and B-cells is diminished, not so much from exhaustion in the output of stem cells as from impaired maturation and specific differentiation, which reduces the population of *reactive* cells. In T-cells this may be attributable to involution of the thymus; in B-cells to deficiencies as yet undetermined. The consequences are that cellular immunity is impaired, delayed-type hypersensitivity responses (e.g. to skin test antigens) are diminished, and there is a rise in serum immunoglobulins (especially IgA and IgG) and autoantibodies.

Besides increasing the incidence of infection, of multiple myeloma, and of giant-cell arteritis, this age-related functional decline is thought to influence or potentiate the appearance of 'diseases of ageing' such as cancer, vascular disease, cerebral degeneration, senile amyloidosis, and maturity-onset diabetes. Welford (1981) suggests that it also mediates the ageing process. He claims that there is a correlation between life span and DNA repair capacity in different species which, in turn, is regulated by the immune system. Therefore, age-related immune dysfunction in a relationship such as this might be supposed to elicit autoimmune responses which would promote a process of active self destruction in the ageing individual.

The genetic component

Most of the theory considered so far suggests *how* ageing may be brought about; *why* it occurs introduces the possibility of genetic determination of longevity. It is not suggested that all the decrements associated with biological ageing are initiated by genes. Some time changes in cell structure and chemistry clearly are not. But if ageing is to be attributed only to a mechanism such as mutation, cross-linkage, error accumulation, or autoimmunity, it must also explain why different species appear to inherit a relatively fixed life span and why it is *species specific* over such a wide range (for example, 1 day for a mayfly, 30 days for a fruit fly, 3 years for a mouse, and 100 years for man). Other evidence suggesting that specific patterns of ageing and death originate in genes is that life span appears to be *sex-linked* in favour of females and, from studies on monovular twins, that *heredity* confers prospects of long life on the children of long-lived parents. The genetic possibilities suggested are:

1 That biological changes of senescence as a prelude to death are programmed in 'ageing genes', the program being played within time determined by a 'biological clock' located in the cell nucleus (Burnet 1970; Hayflick 1976). Thus ageing is conceived as a genetic endowment comparable to growth and development.

2 Senescence is determined in some way by the genetic apparatus but not by specific genes. It is simply 'programmed to run out of programs', and then switch off, much as a tape recorder performs. Development involves differentiation, a gradually increasing repression of genes. The primitive cell can synthesize any specific protein, but differentiated cells, which accumulate with age, are more limited in their protein synthesis and, as vital proteins are increasingly repressed, perhaps cells run out of program and die.

3 The genetic apparatus is programmed for sequential biological events,but not to end the program. This is supposed to occur owing to the kind of error accumulation described earlier which leads to mis-information and intracellular errors.

Burnet (1970) gave the following concise interpretation of genetic and immunological theories of ageing:

1 Ageing in any species is genetically programmed as a result of evolutionary processes.

2 The program is mediated essentially by an inbuilt metabolic clock whose most direct manifestation is the Hayflick limit to cellular proliferation in the euploid state.

3 Organs or physiological systems will differ widely in the time needed to use up their quota of cells. Many systems may never approach the limit but that system, vital to life, which first uses up its quota will be the chief secondary mediator of ageing.

4 Everything points to the thymus-dependent immune system as the key system whose exhaustion is responsible for ageing in mammals and probably other vertebrates.

5 The most essential function of the thymus-dependent system is immunological surveillance: i.e. the capacity to deal with cellular anomaly arising by somatic mutation. These anomalies include cancer and autoimmune disease.

Genetic factors must play a part in ageing, but how they operate is unknown and the cause of the process is a challenge to research not only

in genetics, but in the associated disciplines of virology and immunology.

Physiological theories of ageing
The age-specific decline in faculties which leads to senescence and
death is a fact of life, and its effects on physiological reserves and the
capacity to respond to stress were aptly summed up by Medawar when
he wrote that 'what lays a young man up may lay his senior out'. A
theory of 'wear and tear' to explain this, drawing the analogy with a
machine, is attractive but human mechanisms for self repair are more
advanced than any built into the most sophisticated machines, and the
performance of tissues such as muscle, or physiological functions of
nervous or cardiac systems, can be improved rather than worn down
over most of a healthy lifetime, by practised use or under stress.

When hormones were discovered endocrine theories became popular,
and ageing was attributed to declining function in gonads, thyroid, or
pituitary, but none of these, alone, could account for all aspects of this
complex phenomenon. The pituitary does regulate a vast array of
tissue response throughout the body. Everitt (1981), in a review of this,
maintains that it also regulates the process of ageing and the pathological changes which determine the duration of life. Since the hypothalamus drives the pituitary this involves mediation by the
hypothalmic–pituitary–peripheral endocrine axis, a concept of neuro-
endocrine interaction supported by Shock (1974) from studies of age
changes in the performance of various body systems, and Ordy (1981)
from the investigation of neurotransmitters in the ageing brain. They
believe that whilst the basic cause of ageing may lie at cellular level, the
brain combines with the endocrines as the 'pacemakers of ageing', and
age changes reflect deterioration in the performance and integrative
action of neuro-endocrine control systems.

Hormones are involved in growth, development, and metabolism,
and in the complex autonomic and endocrine mechanisms responsible
for homeostasis, maintaining the constancy of the internal environment
surrounding the tissue cells. The brain plays a unique role in adaptation
to external changes through reflexes, conditioning, and higher forms of
learning. Excitation and conduction in neurons are processed electro-
chemically; transmission across synapses is chemical, involving neurotransmitters and associated enzymes. Therefore, besides the age-related
loss of neuropil and nerve cells, changes in electrical and chemical
activities dependent on neurotransmitters and hormones may be responsible for the decline in sensory function, learning capacity, memory,
motivation, and motor co-ordination in old age and for a breakdown
in control mechanisms. Indeed, with the recent discovery of the pep-

tide hormones of the central nervous system it has been suggested that the brain should now be regarded as an endocrine organ (Stocker 1980).

Physiological research into the process of ageing is less concerned at present with the *cause* than with the *effects*; to dissociate these from disease processes, and to correlate them with chronological age as *indices* of biological or functional age. A reliable index from a battery of such tests will be a better guide than chronological age to administrators and others responsible for the planning of preventive medical and social care, of employment, and of retirement of old agers in the future. However, perhaps the most important aim of this research is to provide the links needed to integrate knowledge across the gap between the minutiae of cell biology and what is known of the physiology of senescence in the whole organism.

Williamson and Johnson (1980) conclude that the process of ageing *may* be the same for all tissues, but they age independently, at their own rate, and on their own program. Secondary ageing may be controlled by a single locus so that all tissues age together but by different processes. Ageing may cause death directly or indirectly in three ways:

1 a decline in the efficiency of the control mechanisms concerned with homeostasis and the ability to cope with stress (as Shock and Ordy suggest)
2 diminished capacity to deal with infection owing to an impaired immunological system, reduced lymphoid tissue (and hence reduced resistance to infection) and declining antibody and hypersensitivity reactions
3 the rising incidence in old age of neoplastic and age-related auto-immune disease (see Burnet 1970)

The application of all this in clinical practice is that in old people evidence of reduced physiological reserves and impaired homeostasis often remains concealed until some form of stress—illness, accident, operation, or toxic condition—tips the balance into failure. This shows up in constellation of symptoms and signs relating to the tissues most at risk, and therefore most affected. The most susceptible, and most likely to be exploited, are those of the central nervous system, those concerned in locomotor activity and in renal function, and those which maintain the equilibrium of the *milieu intérieur*. As examples, mental confusion may dominate the clinical picture of a pneumonia superimposed on impending senile dementia or of dehydration over-taxing impaired renal reserves; acute left-ventricular failure may be precipitated by an adverse drug reaction when inappropriate medication affects an ageing, ischaemic myocardium; minimal stress on osteoporotic bone, even without a heavy fall, may cause a fracture which would not have happened in earlier life.

Effects of ageing

In Table 1 which follows the first column is a list of the morphological changes usually attributed to ageing for different body systems, although they are not necessarily, or not always, without a basis in some pathological process. The second column comprises findings on clinical examination of old people which are usually accepted as 'normal' or inevitable changes imposed by ageing. They may induce the victim, or the relatives, to seek medical help, and may call for sympathetic understanding and appropriate advice, but seldom for investigation or treatment as clinical problems. The third column, with no attempt at detail, shows the more common pathological predispositions of old-agers which do call for medical intervention. This outline is concise, but therefore incomplete, and is no more than a guide to further reading from the bibliography appended.

Table 1. Effects of ageing

Morphological age changes in various systems	Related 'normal' age changes	Clinical pathological trends
Skin		
Atrophy epidermis sweat glands hair follicles	Skin thinned, wrinkled, dry, fragile, and discoloured Greying and recession of hair Nails thin, brittle, ridged, and slow-growing	Abrasions and infections Pruritis; intertrigo Ulcers Onychogryphosis and other nail changes; paronychia
Pigmentary changes	Senile lentigines and seborrhoeic warts	Solar keratoses
Epidermal hyperkeratosis		Carcinoma intraepidermal basal cell squamous cell
Degeneration collagen elastic fibres	Loss of elasticity Senile purpura Campbell de Morgan spots	
Sclerosis of arterioles		
Reduced subcutaneous fat	Less padding Less insulation	Pressure sores Hypothermia
Central nervous system: special senses		
Eye		
Loss of orbital fat	Sunken appearance of eye Laxity of eyelids Senile ptosis	Entropion Ectropion Trichiasis (ingrowing lashes) Basal-cell carcinoma of eyelid
Stenosis of lacrimal duct	Epiphora	Dacryocystitis Lacrimal abscess
Lipid deposits in cornea	Arcus senilis	
Conjunctivitis sicca	Reduced tears; dry cornea	Necrotizing sclerokeratitis; corneal ulcers
		Slow loss of vision
Shallow anterior chamber	Reduced filtration angle Increased intraocular pressure	Glaucoma angle closure (acute) open angle (chronic)
Loss of elasticity and nuclear sclerosis in lens	Presbyopia	Cataract
	Contracted pupils, slowed reflex	Macular degeneration *Sudden loss of vision*
Degenerative changes in muscles of accommodation, iris, vitreous, retina, and choroid	Impaired visual acuity and tolerance of glare Reduced fields of vision Defective colour vision Slowing of dark-adaptation Muscae volentes (objects floating in field of vision)	Retinal detachment Occlusive vascular disease: **1** Central retinal artery or vein **2** Posterior cerebral artery—*cortical blindness* from bilateral occlusion; sometimes denied (Anton's syndrome); visual hallucinations common: pupils react normally. Macular or vitreous haemorrhage

Table 1—*continued*

Morphological age changes in various systems	Related 'normal' age changes	Clinical pathological trends
Degeneration in cortical neurons relating to vision (occipital lobes) and of intrinsic or extrinsic ocular muscles	Visuo-spatial perception and discrimination less accurate Impaired accommodation Limitation of upward gaze	Confusional states caused by sensory deprivation
Ear Degeneration of organ of Corti (loss of hair cells) Loss of neurons in cochlea (ganglion cells) and temporal cortex Impaired elasticity affecting vibration of basilar membrane	Presbyacusis—impaired: 1 Sensitivity to tone (high frequency) 2 Perception (especially against background noise) 3 Sound localization 4 Cortical sound discrimination	Psychological effects of deafness (isolation; suspicion; depression)
Otosclerosis of ossicular chain in middle ear Excessive wax accumulation		Conductive deafness
Atrophy of striae vascularis (impaired endolymph production) Degeneration of hair cells in semicircular canals	Impaired reflex postural control Uncertainty and unreliability in moving about in darkness	Ménière's syndrome
Nose, throat, & tongue Atrophic changes in mucosae Neuronal degeneration (taste buds reduced 64 per cent by age 75) Atrophy and loss of elasticity in laryngeal muscles and cartilages	Impaired sense of taste and of smell Diminished responsiveness of reflex cough and swallowing Vocal folds slack, voice tremulous and pitch raised; power and range reduced	Risks of gas or food poisoning Anorexia Food fads Malnutrition Avitaminosis Sublingual varicosities and haemorrhages Carcinoma of larynx (men) Post-cricoid carcinoma (women)

Central nervous system: brain and spinal cord

Macroscopic changes:

Meningeal thickening, cerebral atrophy (brain weight down 10 per cent between ages 30 and 70)

Table 1—*continued*

Morphological age changes in various systems	Related 'normal' age changes	Clinical pathological trends
Histological changes:		
Earliest is patchy loss of dendrite spines on neurons followed by swelling of dendrite shafts and cell bodies, progressing to fragmentation and cell deaths. (Loss of synaptic connections, impaired electrochemical reactions, and neural dysfunction are thought to follow from reduction in dendrite neuropil (Scheibel and Scheibel 1981)) In all cells—deposits of lipofuscin ('wear-and-tear pigment' formed in degenerating cytoplasm probably from lysosomes or mitochondria) In neurons:	Diminished intellectual responsiveness, mental agility, and abstract reasoning capacity Impaired perception, analysis, and integration of sensory input Failing short-term memory and learning ability Less resilient, more rigid in outlook, tending toward being more self-centred, withdrawn, and introverted	Reduced intellectual reserves predisposing to acute confusional states Dementia—deficits in intellect and memory similar to those of normal senescence begin earlier and act with greater intensity progressing to the disorientation and sustained mental, behavioural, and motor changes of presenile and senile mental deterioration Depression Persecutory symptoms of paraphrenia
1 loss of RNA, mitochondria, and enzymes in cytoplasm **2** Hyaline and eosinophilic inclusions and Lewy bodies **3** Neurofibrillary tangles, senile plaques, and granulo-vacuolar degeneration. Different degenerative changes occurring with increasing frequency in people over 60 years of age, but not directly related with each other Corpora amylacea: occur anywhere in brain tissue	Impaired sensory awareness (of pain, touch, heat, and cold, and joint-position sense) Sensori-motor performance slower to achieve accuracy Impaired mechanisms controlling posture, anti-gravity support, balance, and moving equipoise (nerve conduction velocity reduced 10 per cent by age 75)	Defective appreciation and localization of pain Predisposition to falls and injuries
Vascular changes:		
Intimal and medial fibrosis: Siderosis, amyloid and hyaline degeneration Atheroma—increasing in extent with age, but pathogenesis is multifactorial		Multiple infarct dementia Transient ischaemic cerebral episodes Impending, progressing, and completed strokes Postural instability

Table 1—*continued*

Morphological age changes in various systems	Related 'normal' age changes	Clinical pathological trends
Autonomic nervous system		
Neurotransmission depends on acetylcholine and on the catecholamines dopamine and noradrenalin. Autonomic reflex response is probably weakened in old age by age-dependent reduction in synthesis and hydrolysis of these neurotransmitters combined with receptor loss. Autonomic dysfunction accompanies the Shy–Drager syndrome, parkinsonism, cerebrovascular disease, and various causes of neuropathy, particularly diabetes and alcoholism.	Predisposition to postural hypotension (asymptomatic) Impaired response to Valsalva manoeuvre Diminished baroreflex sensitivity Impaired thermal regulation in response to heat and cold Loss of appreciation of visceral pain Impaired alimentary motility	Symptomatic postural hypotension Defective autoregulation in the cerebral circulation Liability to falls Predisposition to hypo-thermia or heat stroke (p. 70) Misleading presentations of illness (pp. 25 & 30)
Locomotor system *Muscles*		
Atrophy affecting both number and size of fibres conditioned by metabolic disorder and 'functional denervation'.	Loss of muscle bulk Nocturnal cramp Herniae: extra- and intra-abdominal Decline in physical strength—'physiological' weakness Disability, and limitation of range and speed of movements—combined effects of muscular weakness, joint stiffness, and impaired central mechanisms for sensorimotor performance: 1 Less precision in fine movements and in rapid alternating movements 2 Irregular timing of action, loss of smooth flow of one form of action into another 3 Slowing down to avoid outcome of one action before planning the next.	Muscular wasting, especially distal extremities Pathological weakness: 1 Metabolism: deficiency in serum Ca, K, Vitamin D 2 Endocrine: thyrotoxicosis Cushing's syndrome, cortisone myopathy 3 Cardio-respiratory disease, anaemia (anoxia) 4 Carcinomatosis

Table 1—*continued*

Morphological age changes in various systems	Related 'normal' age changes	Clinical pathological trends
Bone loss		
osteoporosis; thinning of trabeculae and enlarged cancellous spaces.	Asymptomatic, or slight backache; kyphosis, stoop and loss of height	Severe backache, kyphosis, and fractures (inadequate bone density) *Osteomalacia*: deficient calcification of normal bone matrix. Bone pain; myopathy; fractures. Paget's disease (osteitis deformans) Bunions; subluxation of small joints in hands and feet Painful feet (and other chiropody problems)
Joints		
Degenerative changes in ligaments, peri-articular tissues and cartilage Synovia are thickened with villous hypertrophy Cartilage becomes yellow and opaque; there may be superficial erosions; and biochemical changes lead to mucoid degeneration; cyst formation and calcification	Loss of elasticity and resilience in joints Stiffness and predisposition to aches and pains Confidence and reliability of activity reduced Difficulty with intricate tasks (especially if complicated by uncompensated visual defect) Stooped posture, loss of height, and other distortions owing to atrophy and effects of weakness in skeleton and major muscle groups responsible for posture and antigravity support.	*Arthritis*: leading to ankylosis and contractures: **1** Osteoarthritis: such a commonplace of old age as to be considered almost 'physiological' **2** Rheumatoid arthritis: a constitutional disorder with onset usually in earlier adult life but not uncommon over 60 in either sex **3** Gout and pseudo-gout **4** Neuropathic arthropathy
Gastrointestinal system		
Dental caries; gingival recession Atrophic changes in jaw	Problems of adaptation to dentures and altered alignment of bite	Retained carious stumps Cysts; dental sepsis Angular fissures Oral ulcers Risk of parotitis Temporo-mandibular arthritis

Table 1—*continued*

Morphological age changes in various systems	Related 'normal' age changes	Clinical pathological trends
Atrophy of mucosae, intestinal glands, and muscularis	Capricious appetite Asymptomatic alterations in intestinal secretion, motility, and absorption occur in 'normal' ageing	Anorexia Malnutrition Hiatus hernia Achlorhydria (incidence increases over age 60): related to defective absorption of iron and vitamins, and to pernicious anaemia
	Constipation (prolonged gastrointestinal transit time) Diverticulosis (anywhere in gastrointestinal tract, but in colon related to a lifetime of low-residue diet)	Dysphagia (pseudo-bulbar palsy: oesophageal reflux, pouches, and carcinoma) Peptic ulcer Faecal impaction Diverticulitis
No significant age changes described in liver, and there are as yet no tests of function sufficiently refined to detect the impairment sometimes suspected in older patients		

Respiratory system

Coalescence of alveoli (atrophy and loss of elasticity in septa) Sclerosis of bronchi and supporting tissues Degeneration of bronchial epithelium and mucous glands	Total lung volume unchanged but vital capacity is diminished, O_2 diffusion impaired and respiratory efficiency reduced; as are sensitivity and efficiency of self-cleansing mechanisms	Increased susceptibility to pneumonia Chronic obstructive airways disease: owing to *emphysema* (which predominates in 'pink puffers') combined with *chronic bronchitis* (underlying 'blue bloaters')
Osteoporosis thoracic vertebrae rib cage Reduced elasticity and calcification of costal cartilage Weakness of intercostal and accessory muscles of respiration	Kyphosis and increasing rigidity of chest wall Functional reserve respiratory capacity is therefore impaired in old age, but clinical evidence is minimal unless evoked by illness. Compliance changes little because the rise to be expected from diminished elastic recoil is offset by increased lung stiffness (fibrosis) and loss of flexibility in chest wall	Pulmonary tuberculosis (reactivation of 'healed' tuberculosis) Carcinoma of bronchus Pulmonary embolism Concurrent respiratory disease and cardiac failure

Table 1—*continued*

Morphological age changes in various systems	Related 'normal' age changes	Clinical pathological trends
Cardiovascular system		
Aorta: loss of elasticity in media and intimal hyperplasia	Aorta dilated and unfolded (may obstruct venous return in left side of neck therefore assess jugular venous pressure on right)	Aneurysm Aortic stenosis Arrhythmias
Cusps of heart valves degenerate: less resilient with nodular sclerosis and sometimes calcification which may extend into interventricular septum	Apex beat difficult to locate if chest rigid or distorted by kyphoscoliosis Stiffened valves cause murmurs: aortic systolic, mitral regurgitant; not necessarily significant	Conduction defects: bundle branch block probably indicates significant heart disease Pulmonary heart disease (pulmonary embolism)
Myocardial changes: lipofuscin deposits, myocardial fibrosis, and amyloidosis Atrophy and fibrosis of media, and intimal hyperplasia in coronary arteries Brown atrophy only in association with debilitating states: malnutrition, cancer, pernicious anaemia, etc. (heart weight correlates with body weight)	No specific age-determined changes or degeneration in the heart (i.e. no 'senile heart disease') can be correlated convincingly with impaired cardiac function in old age but it is accepted that: 1 cardiac output declines owing to reduced stroke volume; 2 therefore capacity for physical work is limited; 3 a given amount of exercise raises heart rate and blood pressure more in old age than in youth.	Blood-pressure changes: difficult to define hyper-tension over age 65. B.P. readings alone do not constitute a diagnosis (it requires evidence of adverse effects on eye, heart, brain, and kidney). Hypotension often more sinister in old age.
Atheroma—incidence increases with age, probably promoted by hypertension and cigarettes	*Mental confusion* and *profound weariness* should raise suspicion of heart disease in old people. They are often more prominent than anginal pain or even breathlessness (because of restricted activity)	Ischaemic heart disease is the most common cause of heart failure in geriatric medical practice

Table 1—*continued*

Morphological age changes in various systems	Related 'normal' age changes	Clinical pathological trends
Genito-urinary system		
Thickening of basement membrane of Bowman's capsule and impaired permeability	Renal efficiency in waste-disposal impaired by reduced renal mass and functional decline:	Renal calculi Renal infections: pyelonephritis, cystitis Prostatic disease
Degenerative changes in tubules	1 The number of nephrons is halved in an average life span	Gynaecological disorders Retention
Atrophy and reduced numbers of nephrons	2 Renal blood flow is also halved by age 75	Incontinence
Vascular changes affect vessels at all levels from intimal thickening of the smallest, to arteriolar hyalinization and intimal hyperplasia in large arteries	3 Glomerular filtration rate and maximum excretory capacity reduced by same proportion. The ageing kidney can still maintain normal homeostatic mechanisms and	
Prostatic atrophy—acini and muscle with focal areas of hyperplasia	waste disposal within limits, but it is less efficient, needs more time, and its reserves	
Benign nodular hyperplasia present in 75 per cent of males over 80 years of age	may be minimal. Therefore relatively minor degrees of dehydration, infection, or	
Histological (latent) prostatic carcinoma demonstrable in most males aged over 90 years (clinical carcinoma very much less)	impaired cardiac output may precipitate failure	

Other sysems

Endocrine
Hormones are maintained at the serum levels required for various homeostatic mechanisms by the balance struck between the rate of synthesis, the rate of secretion, the concentration of specific carrier proteins (which determine the levels of free or active fractions of hormones in circulation), and the rate of metabolic disposal in the tissues. A change in one factor will be offset by a compensatory shift in another to ensure that the hormone blood level remains unchanged. These factors may be affected by ageing (though differently in different systems) but compensation is so effective that serum levels give little indication of age-changes in endocrine function, and they are difficult both to demonstrate and to interpret. Responsiveness and the ability to adapt to changing conditions tend to alter so that, although endocrine failure is not a consequence of normal ageing, it is difficult to distinguish physiological change and, as in other systems, it may be poverty of reserves that precipitates evidence of deficiency.

1 Age does not affect fasting lucose level, but there is an age-related decrease in glucose tolerance. Pancreatic cell secretion in response to hyperglycaemia is diminished, and diabetic abnormality of glucose tolerance increases with age. It is not clear whether this should be attributed to the change in cell sensitivity, to reduced insulin sensitivity (owing to decreased gluco-receptor-response at the cell surface), or to the effects of changing body composition with age, especially obesity. Receptor loss, caused by complex changes in cellular enzyme activity, probably accounts for many age changes in endocrine regulation, but whatever the cause, ageing is acknowledged to be the outstanding factor contributing to clinical diabetes (p. 65).

2 Functional thyroid activity decreases with age; BMR and radio-active iodine uptake fall. The rate of metabolic disposal of thyroxine is probably decreased, and the gland compensates by reducing the secretion rate to keep the hormone blood level unchanged, but there is an age-related fall in plasma levels of triiodothyronine (T_3) converted from thyroxine (T_4). It is not known whether this indicates reduced thyroid production, impaired conversion, or altered disposal rate. The free thyroxine index (serum T_4 divided by T_3 uptake $\times$ 100) and serum TS level are probably the best indices of thyroid performance, but all tests of thyroid function are suspect in old people who are ill. *Myxoedema* is three or four times more common than *thyrotoxicosis* in older people, and atypical presentation is common to both: non-specific debility, anaemia, hypothermia and paranoid psychiatric illness in hypothyroidism; atrial fibrillation unresponsive to digitalis, heart failure, and osteoporosis in hyperthyroidism.

3 A post-menopausal fall in oestrogen levels is associated with an increased rate of loss of bone in elderly women. Primary testicular failure in men over 50 leads to falling plasma testosterone levels and high levels of gonodotrophins. There is increased conversion of androgen to oestrogen in peripheral tissues, declining sexual performance and fertility, and loss of muscle mass.

4 Changes in antidiuretic hormone secretion in the elderly affect responses to haemodynamic stimuli and to serum osmolality and so may induce postural hypotension or upset fluid balance.

Homeostasis
Particularly vulnerable in old age to plasma or blood loss, dehydration, potassium depletion, and metabolic acidosis. At rest the normal old person can maintain a constant internal environment, but capacity to react to stress, even the demands of daily living, is markedly lessened owing to two key characteristics of ageing:

1 poverty of reserve which impairs the ability to restore systematic equilibrium quickly when it is upset:

2 breakdown in co-ordination because different organs age at different rates, and functions dependent on the performance of several systems are therefore impaired.

Age-related shortcomings in neuro-endocrine control mechanisms underlying defective homeostatis have been discussed earlier (pp. 8–9).

2 Essentials of geriatric clinical practice

Implications of an ageing population

It is sometimes suggested that medical science has enabled old people to live longer, creating problems for modern society, but this concept of 'medicated survival' of the elderly is misleading. The increased proportion of old people in the Western world has not been brought about by control of illness in old age. It is the result of control of lethal diseases in childhood, so that many more children now survive to become old, and this is as much a triumph of betterment of social conditions (housing, food, and sanitation) as of advances in medicine. The expectation of life of a male child at birth in Great Britain has increased since 1900 by 22 years (from 48 to 70) compared with only two years (from 13 to 15) for a man of 60. In Canada average lifespan from birth for males increased between 1931 and 1971 from 60 to 70 years, but life expectancy at age 65 only increased from 13·0 to 13·9 over the same period.

The effect of this is to increase the proportion of old people in the community, especially of old women, because their expectation of life is better than that of men by four or five years. This preponderance of women, particularly of very old women, was emphasized by data from the Ukraine showing that their proportion increases at each decade over age 60 until, by 100 years, there are seven times as many women as men. The progressive ageing of the population in Canada is illustrated in Table 2 showing the proportion of old people aged 65 and over at each decade from 1901 to 1972, and comparing the proportion in Canada with other countries in Table 3. It has been estimated that the world population will double in the next 35 years, but the number of people aged 60 and over is expected to double in only 30 years, and the over-eighties are likely to increase by more than 120 per cent.

Morbidity, the rate of illness, rises sharply with each decade after middle life, becoming very high indeed over 70 years of age. These ancients are often the victims of so-called 'degenerative' conditions: cardiovascular, cerebrovascular, renal, or respiratory insufficiency, or of locomotor disorders related to degenerations of the nervous system or

Table 2 Number and percentage of total population aged 65 years and over for Canada 1901–72

Year	Total aged 65+	Per cent aged 65+
1901	271 201	5·1
1911	335 317	4·5
1921	420 244	4·7
1931	567 076	5·6
1941	767 815	6·7
1951	1 086 273	7·8
1961	1 391 154	7·6
1971	1 744 405	8·1
1972	1 787 700	8·2

Table 3 Percentage of total population aged 65 years and over—some comparisons at about 1973

Country	Per cent aged 65+
Africa	3
Asia	3·5
U.S.S.R.	8
United States	10
United Kingdom	13·6

of muscles and joints. Increasing morbidity is therefore associated with increasing rates of mental and physical infirmity and of residual disability after illness (Fig. 1).

In such circumstances an old person inevitably becomes dependent on support of one kind or another from relatives, friends, and social services. Unfortunately, this support is not always forthcoming, and there are several reasons for this.

1 As people grow older they often outlast or outlive their relatives and friends, who themselves are victims of illness and disability. Or the old person who is somewhat eccentric may have withdrawn from contact with the outside world to become a recluse. Very old people readily become isolated for these reasons and their health deteriorates owing to malnutrition, neglect, and apathy.

2 Changing patterns of disease and of need in our ageing communities

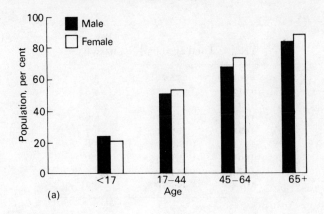

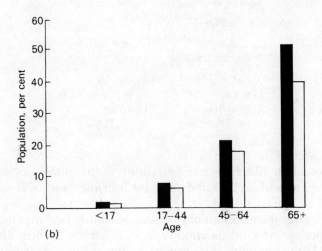

Fig. 1. (a) Percentage of persons with one or more chronic conditions; (b) percentage with limitation of activity (from National Centre for Health Statistics, U.S.A. 1965–6).

in the twentieth century have been accompanied by adverse domestic and social changes creating deficiencies and staff shortages. The deficiencies involve *finance*, in that pensions and supplementary funding never seem able to keep pace with the rising cost of living; *housing*, not only a general lack of homes for old people, but a lack of homes specially designed to meet the needs of the handicapped old-ager; and *preventive care services*, the development and co-ordination of resources needed to support the failing capacities of increasing numbers of old people.

3 It becomes steadily more difficult to recruit the personnel necessary to provide support. In an era when we 'grow three grannies now where we once grew one', the unmarried daughters, aunts, and the family retainers who were once available to look after ageing parents and grandparents are employed full-time today in other activities. Domestic service is no longer a prestigious occupation; the status of nursing and allied professional work is being rivalled by other occupations in business and commerce (with better salaries too); even in nursing, professional idealism and the sense of vocation have waned. Last but not least in this catalogue of difficulties in providing domestic care for the elderly is the fact that more married women go out to work than ever before, so they are not available to provide continuous supervision for an invalid relative.

Hence the demands of ageing populations on health and social services in Western communities which are heavy already must continue to increase. This is evident in the proportions of old people entering hospitals: between 50 and 60 per cent of the admissions to general medical and surgical wards. Recovery is slow, and resettlement in the community prejudiced for those who survive, by residual disability and by these social handicaps. Duration of stay in hospital is unavoidably longer, and even when discharge is successful prolonged follow-up and maintenance services are usually necessary to forestall frequent re-admissions.

Altered patterns of disease in old age

Multiple pathology
In early life the symptoms and signs of illness can usually be explained by a single diagnosis, but in old age, both precise diagnosis as a basis of treatment, and the assessment of disability, are often compromised by the number of active, or inactive, pathological processes affecting the outcome. It has been said that if clinical examination of a sick old person does not reveal at least three or four pathological conditions needing attention, the patient has not been examined properly.

Degenerative and locomotor disorders are pre-eminent in old age: 'degenerative' being a term applied to conditions for which there is no specific treatment because they are of unknown origin, or their pathogenesis is not fully understood. Much geriatric medicine is in this category, but it is constantly being reduced as progress in medicine reveals criteria for the diagnosis of diseases formerly unrecognized, or introduces successful treatment for these or other conditions once thought incapable of an effective response.

The outstanding physical limitations in old age are imposed by *cardiovascular disease*: restricted exercise tolerance in ischaemic heart disease; transient cerebral ischaemia, postural imbalance, and strokes; and intermittent claudication; gangrene, and amputations attributable to peripheral vascular occlusion; *arthritis*: osteoarthrosis or rheumatoid disease; *neuro-muscular disorders* such as parkinsonism, motor neuron disease, and unaccountable muscular weakness and wasting; *cancer;* and the tendency to resistant *pulmonary infections* and *thrombo-embolism*.

Mental disorder in old age still represents the widest field of research opportunity in geriatrics. Any confused behaviour in an elderly invalid used to be labelled 'dementia', implying an irreversible state of mental deterioration. In the past 20 years, a long list of toxic, infective, metabolic, and deficiency states have been recognized as causes of *acute confusion* which responds to appropriate treatment. These and other mental illnesses such as *depression* or *persecutory states*, which may improve with treatment, must be distinguished from the progressive *primary dementias* (e.g. Alzheimer's disease) or the step-wise intellectual decline of recurrent cerebrovascular accidents (multi-infarct dementia), which do not.

Insidious onset

Certain diseases quite common in geriatric medical practice are liable to be disregarded, even by relatives or by a doctor in constant attendance on an elderly invalid, because they develop with slowly progressive changes that are easily missed. Alterations in voice and in facial appearance, cold-sensitivity, lethargy, and slowing up are so gradual, and so easily attributed to 'old age' that *myxoedema* can be overlooked until some observant visitor, who has not seen the patient for a long time, provokes investigation of changes that seem obvious to them. Postural changes, stiffness, and restricted activity are so much a part of ageing that the flexion attitude, bradykinesia, and rigidity of *parkinsonism* may be untreated unless tremor is sufficiently marked to draw attention to it. Dementia, collagen disorders, cancer, or reactivation of pulmonary tuberculosis are other deceptive conditions in geriatric medicine where diagnosis often depends on the use of a good index of suspicion and on being a good noticer: 'able to notice the significance of what, at first sight, is irrelevant' (Asher 1960).

Altered responses to illness
Illness often presents differently in old age than in youth, and textbook descriptions of disease are apt to be misleading when applied in geriatrics.

1 Regulation of the *body temperature* is unstable, or less responsive, so that pyrexia may not be as marked as would be expected even in severe infections such as pneumonia, appendicitis, or pyelonephritis. The converse, a lack of awareness of cold, or of the capacity to react normally to it, may lead to *hypothermia*. Reference has been made earlier to the tendency to *confusion* in geriatric illness and this is often associated with *dehydration* because the patient is not properly aware of thirst and has not been given an appropriate fluid intake. *Water/electrolyte imbalance* develops readily and *constipation* provokes distension and discomfort, adding to the patient's restless and irrational behaviour.
2 Pain sensitivity is diminished and its localization is often capricious in old age. Even in conditions which cause intense pain in earlier life—coronary infarction, pleurisy, peritonitis following a perforated viscus, or a fractured femur—there may be so little discomfort, or it is referred in such bizarre ways, that diagnosis is delayed with fatal consequences.
3 Response to drugs changes with age. Absorption, metabolism, and excretion of certain drugs may be impaired, reducing the patient's tolerance of them, and leading to adverse drug reactions. Digitalis, anticoagulants, hypnotics and sedatives, antidepressants, and anticholinergics are amongst the drugs in common use which are best prescribed and kept under constant review for old people in paediatric rather than adult doses.
4 Recovery from illness is often slow, owing to intercurrent infections (e.g. cystitis or pneumonia), or to debilitating conditions, acquired perhaps from a combination of the medical and social factors mentioned earlier as causes of social isolation and neglect. Healing is retarded in patients whose malnutrition has caused anaemia, protein deficiency, and a lack of vitamin B and ascorbic acid. Without the coenzymes and collagen dependant on these, resynthesis of amino acids and repair processes are delayed. It is often difficult to coax old people to eat after a severe illness, and consideration has to be given to a suitable diet with supplements when necessary.
5 Conversely some old people make remarkable and quite unexpected recoveries from severe mental or physical impairment. It is always necessary to be cautious in prognosis, and to inquire from close relatives

or friends about the patient's mental make-up (motivation and personality) and physical state (range of activity) prior to the onset of illness.

Distinction between disease and disability

Disability has to be recognized and assessed as something apart from disease in old age. Many factors mentioned earlier contribute to it, but it is exaggerated and extended especially by impaired mental capacity, lethargy and weakness, stiffened joints, and loss of postural control and balance. These combine to deprive an elderly invalid of confidence and a sense of security in moving about. If discouragement is allowed to grow and activity to fail the patient finds it easier to stay in bed, exposed then to the added risks of thrombo-embolism, osteoporosis, constipation, bedsores, incontinence, and apathy so well described by Richard Asher (1947):

Look at a patient lying long in bed. What a pathetic picture he makes! The blood clotting in his veins, the lime draining from his bones, the scybala stacking up in his colon, the flesh rotting from his seat, the urine leaking from his distended bladder, and the spirit evaporating from his soul.

Asher concluded his analysis of these dangers and his advice on how to avoid them by taking liberties with *Hymns Ancient and Modern* no. 23, verse 3:

> Teach us to live that we may dread
> Unnecessary time in bed.
> Get people up and we may save
> Our patients from an early grave.

However, the urge to get old people up can be overdone. There are times when a patient, showing no obvious signs of a pathological condition to explain a desire to stay in bed, does indeed have a covert infection, infarction, or metabolic upset which fully justifies reluctance to get up and take exercise, and it is inexcusable to insist that old people who are comatose or approaching death should be required to sit out of bed, tied up for long spells in a chair. It does nothing for them except perhaps add to their miseries. When a patient slumps into a chair, drowsy, incontinent, and unable to hold up his head, one must inquire how long he has been there, and ask why he might not be better supported more comfortably in bed. Insistence on sitting every patient up in a chair regardless of clouded consciousness, discomfort and pain, postural hypotension, and exhaustion is not evidence of intelligent geriatric medical practice. Each patient's needs should be estimated on their merits, and time out of bed should be prescribed and supervised as precisely as any other aspect of treatment.

Unreported disability in old age

The incidence of unreported disabling illness is high amongst old people. They, or their relatives, draw attention to obvious complaints: breathlessness and oedema in heart failure, the effects of a stroke, or the distress of acute respiratory insufficiency. They often fail to report other incapacitating but less dramatic conditions. Musculoskeletal complaints, painful feet, anaemia, urinary infections, and dementia were prominent causes of disability unrecognized by the family and unknown to the patient's doctor in Williamson's survey of people aged 65 and over in three medical practices in Edinburgh (Lowther *et al.* 1970). In a clinic set up to screen old people thought to be at risk of disability from unreported illness the most common disorders found in the first 300 old people investigated were obesity, depression, cataract, deafness, ischaemic heart disease, osteoarthritis, and painful feet. Other covert disorders, less common, but no less disabling, were cervical spondylosis, parkinsonism, vertebral-basilar insufficiency, postural hypotension, osteoporosis and osteomalacia, diabetes, myxoedema, uterine prolapse, carcinoma, pernicious anaemia, hernia, and diverticulitis. The criteria of 'high-risk' old people to be singled out for assessment at such clinics are those who are:

- over 70 years of age
- living alone
- recently bereaved
- disabled by locomotor disorder
- recently discharged from hospital

It is seldom possible to cure much of the illness found by screening clinics, but discomfort can be relieved and the range of independence and interests can be widened for many patients.

Gerontology and geriatrics

Gerontology is the study of the physiology, psychology, and sociology of ageing; *geriatric medicine* is a branch of general medicine concerned with clinical investigation and treatment of the consequences of ageing and its pathological associations. Research interest in the process of ageing and other aspects of gerontology is worldwide, but geriatrics as a clinical discipline was pioneered mainly in Great Britain after the last war, along three lines of development:

1 Limiting the effects of residual disability after illness in old age by a phase of continuing care and rehabilitation, and improving standards of medicine and nursing for chronic and terminal illness. The management and after-care of elderly patients is determined by assessment which depends on four estimates:

a *Diagnosis:* the prerequisite of correct treatment

b *Disability:* assessed and treated independently of the diseases underlying it

c *Mentality:* knowledge of personality, responsiveness, and motivation of the patient prior to the most recent illness indicates what to hope for in recovery

d *Social background:* essential to decisions on resettlement

2 Methods of preventive geriatric care were introduced later to identify the causes of disability in those at risk and to co-ordinate the work of the professionals responsible for geriatric services: administrators, doctors, nurses, therapists, social workers, and the organizers of voluntary action. It is a multidisciplinary group, and all have something to contribute to the betterment of old age. They may work in the community or in institutional settings, but when preventive care in the community fails, and hospital care becomes necessary, it does not matter *how* the patient gets in to hospital but how *readily*.

3 Creating the academic departments necessary to promote education and research. These are the pace-setters of progress and the centres required to attract those with the talent to make it.

Geriatric clinical methods

History-taking and clinical examination have to be modified to meet some consequences of ageing. Students are advised to extend their knowledge within the following outlines by reading an exceptionally good handbook (Caird and Judge 1974) describing techniques of geriatric assessment and variations from conventional clinical methods.

The elderly patient cannot be assessed properly without knowledge of his home circumstances, obtained preferably from a home visit to determine:

1 standards of care and help available at home

2 factors contributing to illness: malnutrition (alcohol); dehydration; neglect and poor habits; adverse drug reactions

3 domestic impediments to resettlement, e.g. stairs after strokes

4 relationships with relatives and friends

5 supporting services: the need; those already in use; availability of others

History-taking
This may be compromised by aged whims and shortcomings.

1 *Time and patience* are needed to allow for deafness, impaired grasp, defective memory, or confusion. Two failings often encountered in old people anxious to be helpful are *confabulation*—inventions to fill gaps in memory—and *gratuitous redundancy* (Critchley 1970)—a garrulous flow of words running on with unnecessary detail, sometimes a feature of dysphasia. However, in spite of the difficulties the patient's story must be considered with care—'listening to what is said, not just hearing'—because in old age, just as in youth, if one listens long enough the patient will often divulge the diagnosis.

2 *Misinterpretation of symptoms:* this may arise owing to altered responses to illness (p. 25), multiple pathology, the range of different illnesses which can present with similar symptoms, and the misleading emphasis given to some of them by old people. For example, difficulty in walking, thought to be caused by arthritis or some peripheral locomotor disorder, may really arise from an intracranial lesion; confusion may be dismissed as 'senile dementia', overlooking the real cause, perhaps pneumonia or dehydration; or weakness may be attributed to 'old age' instead of a medical emergency such as potassium deficiency or myocardial infarction.

The non-specificity of symptoms implies, therefore, that it is often more useful to inquire about a change of activity or of mental and physical capacity, than to try and pin down details of particular symptoms.

3 *Information from other sources* should be obtained about the patient's capacity before the onset of the most recent illness. When a relative or nurse draws attention to changes suggestive of mental or physical deterioration in an old person, however trivial they may seem, due weight should be given to them in a medical assessment. The opinion of someone who knows the patient well, and who has been in close attendance, will often give forewarning of pathological changes before they are confirmed by data from ward charts or laboratory investigations.

Physical examination
Consideration, gentleness, and tact are as important as in paediatric medicine. Co-operation may be limited owing to difficulty in communication caused by confusion or deafness, or to the physical handicaps of arthritis or kyphoscoliosis, or to the apathy and unwillingness of a withdrawn, suspicious old person. Sometimes it is expecting too much of an anxious, frightened, or resentful recluse to submit to undressing for a full 'medical', least of all for such personal indignities as rectal or pelvic examinations. Decisions and empirical treatment may have to be initiated from a provisional diagnosis, and with time and reassurance it may be easier to gain the patient's confidence and co-operation in more thorough examination.

Some of the deviations from the clinical findings expected in earlier life in the different systems are these:

Alimentary system. Symptoms are often misdirected, and blunted appreciation of pain is misleading. Constipation is a commonplace, and diarrhoea is often attributable to faecal impaction. *Vomiting*, however, is always a sinister complaint in old age. Obesity conceals abdominal signs, whereas the thin lax walls of a wasted abdomen fail to develop rigidity with peritoneal irritation, and distend more readily with obstruction. The rectum must always be examined and it is easy, but unforgivable, to miss an obstructed inguinal or femoral hernia.

Respiratory system. Deviation of the trachea is often caused by scoliosis. Chest expansion may be impaired by a fixed bony cage. Chest sounds are often difficult to elicit. It is disturbing to find, with experience, how often a chest radiograph, or post-mortem findings, reveal gross pathological changes in the lungs which were not identified on clinical examination, and this includes massive areas of consolidation.

Cardiovascular system. Pain and dyspnoea are often modified and oedema of the legs (especially asymmetrical oedema) often arises from other causes. Ectopic beats are of little significance in old people. Higher upper limits of blood pressure have to be accepted: over 70 years of age 195/105 for men and 210/115 for women are *not* indications for anti-hypertensive drugs. The apex beat is often difficult to palpate and it is unreliable as an indicator of cardiac size in old people.

Central nervous system. Examination is often difficult because it is made or marred by the ability or willingness of the patient to co-operate. Much of the information required about *mental state* will be noted while taking the history and examining other systems (including the mood, level of consciousness, speech, memory, and behaviour (p. 46)). First impressions of personality are sometimes misleading because the charm assumed for a strange visitor may be quite different from the demanding irritability shown to relatives.

Taste and smell are often impaired in old age; it has to be determined whether deafness is *conductive* (middle-ear disease), *perceptive* (inner ear), *nerve deafness* (eighth nerve or brain-stem lesions), or *central* (impaired comprehension); and there are four retinal changes and causes of impaired visual acuity to be identified: *pigmented* and *haemorrhagic* forms of macular degeneration; *chorio-retinal* degeneration with apparent expansion of the optic disc (as the white choroid shows through a thinning retina): and *diabetic retinopathy* with white or yellow exudates around the macula, micro-aneurysms and haemorrhages. Response to neurological tests is often modified by age (knee jerks are depressed, ankle jerks cannot be elicited, and vibration sense is absent below the knee in many old people). These and other variations to be expected when trying to elicit or interpret neurological signs in old people are considered in more detail by Caird and Judge (1974).

Dependency of ancients

Even with the best of rehabilitation and preventive care services our society cannot evade the responsibilities of a rising rate of dependency in very old people. This might be called 'essential' or 'unavoidable' dependency. Mentally alert and responsive, and without any specific illness to account for their infirmities, these ancients are frail, unsteady, and unreliable in their activities, and in their capacity to look after themselves. They may help with their dressing, bathing, and toilet care, and with cooking, cleaning, and maintaining their homes, but being unable to go out of doors unassisted, they lose contact with shops, church, and other outside interests. They live *precarious* lives, constantly at risk of injury or illness, which, though of minor significance in itself, may precipitate a major crisis for an old person living alone. The proportion of these old-agers grows steadily and their problems make special demands on a doctor's knowledge and intelligent use of social service resources and skills.

Preventive geriatric care

In most countries many *statutory* services are available to reinforce the domestic care of infirm old people or of those in terminal illness. They include nursing, visiting, help in the home, delivery of meals, transport, night sitters, laundry, bathing, and chiropody. *Voluntary* resources include regular friendly visiting, clubs and outings. Both services supply essential equipment of one kind and another—lifting aids, special chairs, bedding, commodes, and other nursing and disability appliances. To relieve hard-pressed relatives, short-term admission can be arranged to a geriatric unit or residential home and most areas have holiday and boarding-out schemes and services for those handicapped by blindness, deafness, or amputation. There are dwellings designed especially for the aged, or help can be given to reconstruct and adapt an existing home to meet disability.

These services have grown to meet a need evident in the fact that 95 per cent of people aged 60 and over live either in their own or in relatives' homes, and it is here that the demand for preventive geriatric care, and often for terminal care, is greatest. Facilities may vary between urban and rural areas, or between one county and another, but they are widely available, and only when they prove to be inadequate should the alternative of institutional care be considered. This may be forestalled for many months, even with heavily dependent invalids, when institutional resources can be extended into the community. If no medical or nursing attention is needed, a *day centre* may accept responsibility for part or all of the working day for an invalid who might otherwise be a source of constant anxiety at home owing to physical, or more often, mental frailty. More heavily handicapped patients may need the daytime cover and specialized services of a geriatric or psychiatric *day hospital*.

Day care such as this is an invaluable component of preventive geriatric medicine. Assessment of disease and disability is made possible without admission; confidence is established between patient, relatives, family doctor, and those responsible for care services; incipient breakdown in an old person, or in precariously balanced home conditions, can be anticipated and prevented; and immediate admission to familiar surroundings under the care of well-informed staff can be assured.

These resources are only as effective as the professions using them are themselves efficient. Their value to the elderly (and even more to their relatives) is proportionate to the skill and experience of a health visitor, who, attached to a group general practice, for example, provides the links between family doctor, patient, social services, and hospital. The 'at risk' patients in the practice are known to her and are listed for regular visits and for the liaison necessary to devise appropriate preventive care. Deteriorating conditions are referred to the family doctor who may arrange an assessment visit from a geriatric physician or request admission to hospital. Here a medical social worker becomes responsible for first-hand knowledge of personalities and home conditions, and for subsequent arrangements for resettlement and aftercare.

Geriatric medical social work calls for tolerance and sympathy with the eccentricities and failings of old people, and for a sound knowledge of local statutory and voluntary resources. A social worker's special contributions are to act as counsellor to anxious and often muddled old people, to their relatives, and to their medical advisers, and, by the reliability of her assessments, to inspire confidence in those who consult her, particularly the matrons of residential homes and the wardens of sheltered accommodation. They often come to depend on her advice for prospective admissions or discharges, and together they can help an old person to gather fading remnants of dignity and to give them at least an illusion of deciding their own destinies.

Utopian health and social services would have solutions to all medical–social problems of old age. Unfortunately even the most considerate and well-informed doctor, medical social worker, or health visitor, however anxious to do their best on behalf of an ageing invalid, must accept that increasing demand conflicts with limitations imposed by economic constraints, cuts in essential services, and reduced staff to operate them.

It is appropriate to conclude this chapter with the reminder that the enlightened medical, nursing, and social services available to society today were subsidized in their development by the working lives of the older generation in hard times. No matter how tiresome their complaints, anxieties, or frustrations in illness may seem, the professional care they demand is their due, and it should be given with consideration, compassion, and, above all, with good manners.

3 Common complaints in old age

DISORIENTATION—DELIRIUM—DEMENTIA

Disorientation

'Orientation' in a clinical sense includes a person's awareness of time and place in relation to himself and others, the recognition of personal friends and familiar places, and the ability to remember at least some past experience and to register new data. It is dependent, therefore, on ability to recall learned memories and to make effective use of memory.

'Disorientation' with failure to appreciate what time it is, where one is, or to recognize relatives or friends, is a common feature of organic brain damage. It may be possible to demonstrate also more subtle forms of disorientation in some patients who are unable to orientate themselves properly in space, or who have lost their sense of body-awareness and fail to identify their own body segments in proper relation to one another.

Correct orientation is synonymous with 'full consciousness', being fully aware of whereabouts and what is going on, and disorientation usually occurs in association with either clouded consciousness or the progressive memory impairment characteristic of advancing dementia. 'Consciousness' is difficult to define because its nature is not fully understood.

Neurology lends support to the distinction between the content of consciousness and the state of consciousness itself. The content of consciousness consists of sensations, emotions, images, memories, ideas, and similar experiences, and these depend upon the activities of the cerebral cortex and the thalamus and the relations between them, in the sense that lesions of these structures alter the content of consciousness without as a rule changing the state of consciousness as such. On the other hand, recent work has shown that other structures, particularly that part of the central reticular formation of the brain stem, which is known as the ascending reticular activating system and which extends at least from the lower border of the pons to the ventromedial thalamus profoundly influence the state of consciousness [Walton 1977].

Drugs which tend to produce unconsciousness selectively depress this system; others which cause wakefulness facilitate it.

Elderly patients who are disorientated are often referred to as being 'confused'. This overworked term covers a wide range of eccentricities of speech and behaviour and should not be applied as if it were a diagnosis. It may apply to a patient with the memory loss of early *dementia*, forgetful, disorientated, and wandering; to the retarded, dejected old person with *depression*; to the patient whose consciousness is clouded in the *delirium* of acute illness; to the delusional *paranoia* of late-onset schizophrenia; or even to the dysphasia and incoherence so common in the hemiplegic recovering from a stroke.

Allison (1962) listed three principal clinical pictures of mental disturbance which present in old people with organic brain disease:

1 acute or subacute states of mental confusion occurring in apparently previously healthy persons, in whom the symptoms are related to gross disturbances of consciousness

2 chronic amnesic syndromes, in which the chief feature is impairment of memory and intellect. In these patients there is usually some clouding of consciousness, but this is never so apparent as it is in the first group

3 patients with neurological signs indicative of focal cerebral disease, e.g. hemiparesis, hemianopia, dysphasia, in whom symptoms of (1) and (2) are superimposed

Transient or protracted, episodes of clouding of consciousness are especially common in old age and may be the first indication of the presence of an organic mental disorder. As they are potentially reversible their recognition is important in deciding both the degree of intellectual and behavioural abnormality, and the appropriate treatment.

Delirium

Acute confusion or acute brain syndrome is a common effect on brain function of physical illness in old age. There is a wide range of causes within the following groups:

Trauma: concussion; subdural haematoma; fat embolism; burns; anaesthetics; operations

Infection:
  a *acute:* throat; chest; genito-urinary
  b *chronic:* tuberculosis; diverticulitis; syphilis

Infarction: cerebral; cardiac; pulmonary; hypotension; heart failure

Toxic: adverse drug reaction; alcohol; carbon monoxide; dehydration; uraemia; hepatic failure

Deficiencies and metabolic upsets:
    a *acute:* hypoxia; haemorrhage; hypoglycaemia; hypothermia
    b *chronic:* anaemia; malnutrition; malabsorption; water/salt imbalance

General diseases: arteritis; neoplasm; diabetes; hypo- and hyperthyroidism

The following is a convenient checklist of causes of acute delirium (J. P. Gemmell):

1 *Drug ingestion*
2 *Infection* (gram-negative septicaemia): chest; genito-urinary; acute cholecystitis
3 *Renal/electrolyte disorder:* dehydration; hyponatraemia (diuretics); azotaemia
4 *Hypoxia:* cardiac failure; pulmonary infection; obstructive lung disease

    Other causes of restless behaviour (especially at night) to be included are:

1 *Deprivation:* hunger; thirst
2 *Discomfort:* cold, damp bedding (incontinence); urinary retention; faecal impaction; paraesthesiae; cramps; unidentified pain; persistent cough
3 *Anxiety:* loneliness, apprehension; lack of security; real or imaginary worries; depression

Special points
1 The delirious patient is usually wakeful, restless, rambling, often hallucinated or deluded, noisy, and behaves irrationally, i.e. 'disturbed and disturbing'.
2 Confusion in patients with no previous history of mental impairment is attributable to cerebral causes (usually cerebral infarction) in one third, and to extra-cerebral causes (most often heart failure, pneumonia, uraemia, anaemia, and hepatic failure) in one half.
3 Transient confusion provoked by a slight or trivial physical disturbance suggests that a latent dementia is being brought to light (poverty of reserve in a deteriorating cerebral cortex).
4 Drugs which induce mental disturbance are:
    a antihypertensives

b diuretics and digitalis
c sedatives and 'neuroleptics': barbiturates, bromides, primidone, amitryptyline, diphenhydramine, diazepam, haloperidol, lithium carb., reserpine, phenothiazines, narcotics, propoxyphene, pentazocine, anticholinergics, levadopa, amantidine

Drug-induced mental disorder presents in two forms:
a agitated confusion, hallucination, altered personality, emotional lability; or
b withdrawal, retardation, memory deficit, disorientation.

Either may be attributed, in error, to dementia in an old person.

Dementia

'Dementia', implying progressive intellectual decline, may develop as a feature of many diseases. In this sense it is not in itself a diagnosis, but defined as sustained intellectual deterioration with mental, behavioural, and motor changes, the term applies particularly to the degenerative and arteriopathic forms:

1 *Degenerative:*
  a pre-senile:
    i   Alzheimer–Pick
    ii   Jacob–Creutzfeldt
    iii   Huntington's chorea
  b senile dementia
  c Parkinson's disease
2 *Arteriopathic* (multi-infarct dementia):
  a atherosclerotic
  b lacunar state (hypertension)
  c giant-cell arteritis

Almost all dementia in old people arises from one or other of these groups—about 50 per cent is degenerative, most of it the Alzheimer pattern of pre-senile or senile cerebral change; 20 per cent is arteriopathic, disintegration of intellectual faculties related to multiple infarction in cerebrovascular disease; and another 20 per cent is a mixture of both. Dementia complicating other disorders accounts for the small proportion remaining; they are important in diagnosis because the mental state may improve with response to treatment of the underlying condition:

1 *Space-occupying lesions:* head injury or subdural haematoma; cerebral tumour or abscess; normal pressure hydrocephalus
2 *Toxic:* drug misuse; alcohol (hepatic failure, cardiopathy); carbon monoxide

3 *Nutritional:* malnutrition; malabsorption (pernicious anaemia); avitaminosis (vitamin B complex)
4 *Metabolic:* thyroid disease; hypoglycaemia; electrolyte imbalance

Other possibilities are infections (bacterial, viral, or *neurosyphilis*) especially with an unsuspected abscess; hypoxic states; and hypercalcaemia (subclinical osteomalacia).

The search for treatable conditions, especially in dementia of rapid or sub-acute onset, may necessitate hospital admission for full investigation including radiography, EEG, and computerized axial tomography.

Aetiology
The cause of senile dementia is unknown, and its pathogenesis remains obscure. Despite analysis of a vast accumulation of data from electron microscopy, molecular biology, neurochemistry, genetics, virology, and immunology, it is still not known whether senile dementia is a distinct pathological disease process, or simply represents an exaggerated form of normal age change.

Cortical atrophy is marked, with much-dilated lateral ventricles; histologically there is marked proliferation of *senile plaques* (aggregations of granular or filamental fragments, with a dense core and amyloid deposits), and of Alzheimer's *neurofibrillary tangles* (bundles of abnormally thickened fibres twisted into crescentic, triangular or circular shapes). Nerve cell loss and intracellular pigment accumulations greatly exceed the normal age change. Granulovascular degeneration in neurons in some areas and amyloid congophilic angiopathy have been described. Neurochemical studies have shown reduced levels of the enzymes concerned with cholinergic neurotransmission and other neurotransmitter systems may also be involved, suggesting the possibility of a chemical means to arrest or reverse intellectual decline. There is no evidence yet to support belief in transmissible slow virus encephalopathy as the cause of senile dementia; it is possible that immune deficiency or autoimmune disease may play some part.

Characteristics
Senile dementia (chronic brain failure). Senile dementia follows a fairly regular path (Godber 1975), from an insidious onset through a course of remorseless intellectual decline:

1 *Mental changes:*
  a Forgetfulness—problems with cooking, money, and shopping; disappearing out of home and getting lost; unable to dress; failing personal hygiene; incontinence; habits deteriorating; getting lost even at home; failure to recognize relatives or friends

b Impaired grasp: loss of capacity for learning and abstract thought
c May be moody and irritable or placid and contented
d Disordered speech—either a poverty of speech progressing to mutism, or disintegration of language to incoherent mumbling jargon
e Loss of humour—humour is 'surprise of the unexpected' and the dementing person has no longer the mental agility to change gears fast enough to appreciate a joke (Mahler 1975)

2 *Behavioural changes:*
   a slower, more rigid thinking
   b becomes withdrawn and self-centred
   c loss of affection
   d eats less: weight loss; frequent cat-naps; restless, aimless wandering

3 *Motor changes* More apparent in later stages
   a stooped posture
   b bradykinesia with slow hesitant movement (may be mistaken for parkinsonism)
   c liability to fall—forward or backwards
   d apractic gait

4 *On examination:*
   a resistance to passive movement (*gegenhalten*—'holding against')
   b loss of ability to move eyes without turning the head
   c motor impersistence—cannot keep eyes closed, tongue out, or maintain a fixed gaze in a given direction
   d grasp, snout, and palmo-mental reflexes often positive, and also the glabellar tap sign

Multi-infarct dementia. This develops at an earlier age than senile dementia, usually with a history of major or minor strokes, and affects more men than women. There is step-wise deterioration in mental capacity following successive cerebrovascular episodes, but the patient often retains the insight that is lost early in senile dementia, and is distressed by the awareness of his condition and by the lachrymose emotional incontinence that often goes with it. Dysphasia or dysarthria and focal pyramidal signs may be more prominent than in senile dementia, with pseudo-bulbar palsy, pareses, increased reflexes, extensor plantar responses, and disorders of posture, balance and gait (p. 48).

About one person in ten aged 65 and over has dementia (Kay, Beamish, and Roth 1964) rising almost to one in four of those aged 80+, and for every demented patient looked after in hospital five are cared for at home. Doctors, nurses, and social workers should be on the watch for signs of dementia in their older patients to ensure in the early stages the effective control of restlessness, nocturnal rambling, or aggression in the patient, and the counselling and support from social and institutional services that are likely to be needed by relatives and neighbours.

Table 4 Differential diagnosis of dementia

	Similarities	Differences
Depression	Apathy; unresponsiveness; memory loss; self-neglect; incontinence of urine	Often recent and acute onset; memory loss patchy and fluctuates day to day; says: 'I don't know' in response to questions; shows distress; family and previous history; response to treatment
Toxic confusional states	Confusion; disorientation; self-neglect; incontinence of urine	Recent, acute onset; clouding of consciousness; drowsiness fluctuates; lucid periods; hallucinations
Paraphrenia	Impairment of thinking; emotional flattening; apathy; delusions	Memory and intellect intact, hallucinations; primary delusions; feeling of passivity
Dysphasia (tumour or stroke)	Talks nonsense; appears confused	Rapid onset; focal neurological signs; clouding of consciousness; focal fits

Reproduced by kind permission from Exton-Smith and Overstall (1979)

CEREBROVASCULAR DISEASE—STROKES— MENTAL BARRIERS TO RECOVERY

Cerebrovascular disorders

The pathogenesis of cerebrovascular disease is considered in detail elsewhere (Adams 1974*a*) with appropriate references. The main points are:

1 Lesions of the intra-cranial vessels are always considered in relation to the cerebral circulation as a whole, taking proper account of the large vessels in the neck, the extracranial component, and of cardiac efficiency in maintaining an adequate head of blood pressure.
2 Collateral safeguards of the cerebral circulation are recognized to be much more extensive and even more efficient than were supposed.

3 Collateral circulation is impaired either by disorders which are *extrinsic* to the blood vessels, such as cervical spondylosis, with associated disc degeneration and exostoses, or *intrinsic*, such as congenital anomalies and arterial diseases, especially atheroma. When many vessels are abnormal, blood flow in the territory of some may be reduced to such precarious levels that even very slight changes in the constancy of the supply, or of its composition, may diminish circulation or oxygenation of the dependent parts of the brain below critical minimal need. This is the state of impending cerebral ischaemia described as 'cerebral vascular insufficiency' (Corday *et al.* 1953). 'Thus although a man is as old as his arteries he is as young as his collateral circulation will permit' (Allison 1964).

4 Atheroma is the main cause of the complex alterations in blood flow brought about by distortion of blood vessels, by intimal damage initiating thrombosis or haemorrhage, or by the release of platelet microemboli. Investigation of blood flow has progressed from the early studies of the properties of blood vessels and linear flow in them, to estimates of total blood flow, and later of regional blood flow, until research is now focused on the physical, biochemical, and pharmacological responses of the micro-circulation in life. This involves cerebral angiography, isotope brain scanning, computerized axial tomography, and other sophisticated techniques of investigation.

5 The nervous system is easily the most sensitive indicator of disordered function anywhere in the body (Bedford 1959) because:

a The brain is less able than other body organs to withstand metabolic deprivation.

b The brain is heavily dependent on the efficient performance of other systems: respiratory, cardiovascular, renal, hepatic, endocrine, and haemopoietic. Its physiological reserves and the mechanisms of autoregulation of cerebral blood flow ensure that its metabolic needs are met with constancy and reliability. Old age, the pathological changes of Alzheimer's disease, or ischaemic brain damage in cerebrovascular disease all may cause loss of neurons and disordered neurochemistry in the particular systems. Evidence of this cell loss or cell damage may appear as symptoms and signs of functional deficit relating to the systems most affected. Sometimes this clinical evidence does not appear until some form of stress, perhaps no more than some mental effort, physical exertion, or a minor illness, makes demands on the deteriorated area of brain tissue which it can no longer meet.

6 When collateral supply and fail-safe systems are eroded to an extent which leaves the brain in this state, it is at the mercy of even slight impairment or imbalance of factors only indirectly related to the cerebral blood supply. These factors can elicit signs of disordered cerebral function of a kind which depends on the area of brain most susceptible to the adverse effects they induce, although this may be remote from the apparent source of the trouble.

Many variables, described as 'ischaemia modifying factors' (Adams 1958) may act singly or together to produce such symptoms. They include disorders which cause alterations in:

a blood flow in the extracranial circulation: changes in blood pressure or arrhythmia effecting cardiac output; kinks, narrowing, or intravascular causes of reduced flow in large vessels

b oxygen-carrying capacity of the blood: respiratory insufficiency, anaemia

c blood chemistry: glucose; water/electrolyte imbalance; acid–base equilibrium; blood lipids

d thrombogenic or thrombolytic properties

e viscosity: platelet aggregation and adhesiveness

Hence, although many old people appear to be in excellent health because they have good hearts and collateral circulations, they are, none the less, fragile. Preservation of the constancy of their *milieu intérieur* is precarious, and they should be labelled 'handle with care' (Allison 1964). This is confirmed in a recent review (Adams 1979) of the abnormal haemodynamics and the pathophysiology of ischaemic brain damage in old people, and of the variations in neurological and intellectual disability associated with it.

Strokes

A stroke is *an acute disturbance of cerebral function of presumed vascular origin with disability lasting more than 24 hours.* It is not to be regarded as an isolated event or diagnostic entity, but should be considered in proper perspective against brain damage in general, and against vascular brain damage in particular. A stroke is only one of four main presentations of cerebrovascular disease, and not necessarily the most important. The others are transient ischaemic episodes, disorders of postural fixation and balance, and dementia.

The pathogenesis, diagnosis, and treatment of acute cerebrovascular accidents at onset are covered in detail in textbooks, and routine investigation of elderly patients with established stroke, and indications for further detailed neurological investigation, with special reference to the value of the scintiscan, and computerized tomography, have been described by Caird (1979). Some points need emphasis here:

1 At least 20 per cent of patients with cerebral vascular accidents have ischaemic heart disease as well, and it is essential always to exclude

myocardial infarction or arrhythmia as added complications of strokes.
2 About 7 per cent of cerebral tumours present as hemiplegia of sudden
onset, and strokes attributable to vascular disease can appear gradually
with headache and a slow ingravescent progression of signs.

Even with the best use of modern investigative techniques, the differential diagnosis of a cerebral tumour from a vascular lesion may only be
decided by *time* and systematic *reassessment*, but the distinction is of
practical, not academic importance. A patient with a cerebral tumour
should not be expected to make efforts to comply with a rehabilitation
programme that is beyond his failing capacities; whereas the patient
making a painfully slow recovery from a vascular lesion must not be
denied the unremitting efforts needed to avoid being discarded pre-
maturely as an incurable chronic invalid.

Effects of strokes, in patients who survive the critical early stages,
show progress towards recovery, however slight, in the following weeks.
If this progress is not being made within 48 hours, or if incongruous
signs, especially fits or involuntary twitching develop, suspicions should
be aroused provoking a search for causes of delayed recovery including:

- head injury sustained at the time of apoplexy
- cerebral oedema
- space-occupying lesion: subdural haematoma; tumour; abscess
- hypothermia or hyperpyrexia
- respiratory complications: pneumonia, hypo- or hyperventilation
- injudicious medication: especially morphine, chlorpromazine, insulin
- electrolyte imbalance and uraemia
- renal tract and other infections
- cardiac infarction and arrhythmia
- associated disease: anaemia; giant-cell arteritis; bacterial endocar-
  ditis; diabetes; polycythaemia
- epilepsy developing after a stroke
- extending cerebral infarct or haemorrhage; recurrent embolism

The following two conditions deserve special reference because they
are not uncommon and both may respond well to appropriate treatment:

1 Stroke patients are at risk of hypothermia because the onset is often
early in the morning and the patient, collapsing after getting out of
bed feeling unwell, may be uncovered for some hours on the floor before
being found. Increasing lethargy and apathy develop as the immobile
body temperature falls, the patient becomes disorientated and de-
tached below 35 °C, consciousness is lost at 30 °C (and this may be

attributed erroneously to the stroke), and cardiac arrest occurs below this level.

2 The conspicuous features of giant-cell arteritis are the *dejection*, the *diversity* of associated symptoms, the progressive *deterioration* (and the risk of blindness in cranial arteritis), and the *high erythrocyte sedimentation rate*. It may present as an indeterminate debilitating illness easily attributed to 'old age' or 'rheumatism' with or without low-grade fever, malaise, anorexia, vague aches and pains, weakness, and loss of weight; or these constitutional symptoms may be overshadowed by the intense headache and tender, inflamed temporal or occipital vessels of *cranial (temporal) arteritis*, or by the girdle pains and weakness of the large muscles of shoulders and hips in *polymyalgia rheumatica*. The importance of early diagnosis and immediate steroid treatment cannot be over-emphasized. The condition is a medical emergency because there is a high risk at any time of an ischaemic lesion causing sudden blindness, hemiplegia, coronary infarction, or some other disaster which is easily prevented by the quick and effective response to steroids. Treatment with prednisone (30 mg daily) should be started, *without* diagnostic arterial biopsy or other investigative delay, in an elderly patient presenting with a constellation of symptoms such as this, otherwise unexplained, and accompanied by a raised erythrocyte sedimentation rate. Usually the rapid response, with an improved sense of well-being, relief of symptoms, and a fall in the sedimentation rate, is itself diagnostic. Prolonged maintenance with prednisone (5–10 mg daily) may be necessary to prevent relapse. If there is little immediate improvement the diagnosis must be reconsidered, and the prednisone may have to be tapered off.

The notes that follow refer mainly to residual disability in the survivors of strokes, a subject of importance if only because of its impact on health and welfare resources. The annual incidence of strokes in Western communities is just less than 2 per 1000 of population, rising with age, especially amongst women. In a population of 250 000 this is equivalent to about 500 new strokes each year. Of these about 250 die early, 50 need continuing care for total disability, and 150 survive with moderate to severe handicap, the remainder being only slightly disabled. The average survival time of these victims will be about $3\frac{1}{2}$ years, so that the prevalence of disabled survivors is considerable.

Points in management
1 The patient cannot be expected to have a better mental or physical performance after a stroke than before it; therefore it is necessary to have an estimate of former capacity.

2 No two hemiplegics are alike; therefore patterns of care in a re-habilitation programme must be flexible, designed to meet individual needs.

3 Emphasis in management is on remaining ability and reserves, i.e., on *capacity* not on disability. The tendency of many stroke victims is to bewail their losses, and much painstaking effort is necessary from those responsible for rehabilitation to turn their attention towards remaining assets and not to commiserate too much on what has been lost; con-gratulate the patient rather on what he has left.

4 Select patients for rehabilitation by criteria of acceptance *not* by defining criteria for rejection. However, resources are limited and should not be expended in vain attempts to rehabilitate a known 'loser', for example a patient with long-standing dementia. This may appear to be obvious, but it is often overlooked when the patient's previous history and abilities have not been investigated thoroughly. Confident prediction about prospects can seldom be given under *12–16 weeks*, and the ultimate grade of recovery may be uncertain for *24 or 30 weeks*. Maximum recovery from major stroke often takes *2 years*.

5 Failure to thrive demands an explanation. It is essential to develop a sensitive index of suspicion for incongruous signs in the course of the illness, and, as in acute strokes, to search for causes of delayed recovery in: (a) a review of diagnosis; (b) a search for associated disorders.

This calls for a means of systematic assessment which, in hemiplegic patients, includes an estimate of *capacity*, essential for several reasons:

  a to determine the patient's prospects and prognosis

  b to assess the patient's needs, to design a programme of treatment appropriate to them and to the estimated 'rehabilitation potential'

  c as an index of the effectiveness of treatment:

   i to gauge individual progress

   ii to compare progress in one patient with another

   iii to compare groups of patients

  d as a basis for standard rating scales for national and international comparisons

There are no agreed criteria of assessment available yet. When defined they should indicate what the patient actually says or does on examina-tion, avoiding non-specific terms such as 'confused', 'dementing', or 'inco-ordinated', to describe the response to tests. What the patient says he can do, and what he does may be quite different things.

Tests of capacity, mental and physical, are described elsewhere (Adams 1974a). In applying them allowances must be made, for *de-fective communication* in deaf or dysphasic patients, for *loss of recent memory*, and for the *inattentiveness* of a patient whose consciousness is still clouded.

Assessment

Six criteria of assessment are suggested:

1 *Exercise tolerance:* strength and endurance within limits imposed by associated diseases (senile weakness, arthritis, cardiac or respiratory insufficiency, amputation, or other locomotor disorders)

2 *Motivation:* necessitating inquiries from relatives about personality and make-up prior to the stroke

3 *Mental capacity:*
  a appearance and mood
  b level of consciousness: comprehension, concentration, insight, orientation, perseveration
  c speech: receptive or expressive dysphasia
  d memory: immediate, recent, and past
  e behaviour: initiative, spontaneity, continence, emotional state
  f performance: self-care, reasoning, apraxia, catastrophic reactions

4 *Motor deficits:*
  a extent and severity of spasticity (or persistent flaccidity)
  b postural abnormality, involuntary movements, contractures
  c degree and distribution of returning voluntary power

5 *Sensory deficits* (perception is assessed before mental capacity):
  a eye
  b ear
  c proprioception
  d discrimination

6 *Postural control:* see below

Recovery of enough independence to get up, to dress, and to move about unaided may be the most that many hemiplegics can hope for by way of recovery, but may mean everything to their morale. The essentials in rehabilitation are emphasis on normal postural settings and patterns of movements rather than on muscle strengthening; on sensory input and awareness of activity in hemiplegic limbs; and on initiation of movements from proximal muscle groups (Adams 1974*a*; 1976).

Uncomplicated recovery seldom presents problems, and a pattern of treatment is usually straightforward. *Delayed recovery* is usually attributable either to defects of higher mental or integrative function which have been called 'mental barriers' to recovery from strokes, or to disorders of posture and balance.

Mental barriers

There are four groups:

1 *Inability to learn.*
   a clouded consciousness
   b aphasia
   c memory defect
   d dementia

2 *Disturbed perception.* Attitudes to illness are disordered by separation from reality.
   a anosognosia ('without knowledge of disease')
   b neglect (of hemiplegic limbs)
   c denial (of illness or of ownership of paralysed limbs)
   d disordered spatial orientation

Body image or body scheme (Head and Holmes) denotes conscious appreciation of the relationship between different parts of the body in space. There is thought to be a representation of the properly integrated body segments on the parietal cortex, and sensory input of joint-position sense and of proprioceptive sensation are constantly matched against this. Disorders of the integrative process result in a form of agnosia (loss of awareness for example of body-half, or of disease—anosognosia).

3 *Disordered integrative action.*
   a loss of postural fixation
   b apraxia: inability to initiate a familiar pattern of voluntary movement in the absence of a motor, sensory, or co-ordination deficit to account for it
   c agnosia: a failure of intellectual recognition (i.e. at cortical level) although the elements of primary identification are intact (the sensory input from eye, ear, or discriminative sensation)
   d perseveration: continuation of a purposeful response which is more appropriate to a preceding stimulus than to the succeeding one which has just been given
   e synkinesia: associated movements; involuntary movements of synergic muscle groups accompanying the voluntary movements of a hemiparetic limb or involuntary movements of imitation in one limb accompanying voluntary movements of the other

4 *Disturbed emotion.*
   a emotional instability
   b apathy
   c loss of confidence; fear
   d unwillingness to try

e catastrophic reaction: a change from amiable co-operation to agitated irritability
f depression

There are two special points to remember about these mental barriers:

1 the hemiplegic patient seldom has the insight to complain about them and attention is drawn to them usually by an observant nurse, relative or therapist who notices incongruous behaviour or lack of response
2 recognition of these defects is of practical importance because unless they are identified appropriate treatment to find some way around them cannot be devised

Postural control (see also next section)
'Posture accompanies movement like a shadow' (Sherrington)
'All movements start from and end in posture' (Keele and Neil 1973)
The mechanisms of postural control are complex and we are liable to forget the extent of practised skills involved in walking, especially when dealing with a hemiplegic patient who is trying to relearn them. An outline of the physiology of walking and disorders of gait are discussed in the next section.

CONTROL OF POSTURE—DIFFICULTY IN WALKING — FAINTS AND FALLS

Control of posture

Man is born with the neurological systems needed to stand and walk but needs time to learn to use them. Steppage movements can be elicited by supporting a new-born infant on its feet, but the mechanisms of antigravity support, postural function, and control of equilibrium are not fully developed (e.g. myelination of the pyramidal neurons is incomplete) and the child needs some years of practice before being able to synchronize them with instantaneous, unthinking accuracy in skilled precision movement. Walking is this kind of learned skill. It entails the postural control and balance necessary to support the body weight in the forepart of each foot in turn, shifting the centre of gravity from side to side, and forward, but always controlled in equilibrium, as the arms swing, and the trunk sways, to counterpoise the swinging leg and maintain the necessary propulsion. Physical make-up, posture, and timing are combined with years of experience throughout childhood to establish the learned memories underlying the ability to walk, or to perform even more intricate patterns of movement such as those involved in skating or hitting a fast-moving tennis ball. Each individual develops a personal level of proficiency, some more polished, more flowing, than others, and some leading athletes become very good indeed. The variety of grace and awkwardness dependent on personal make-up and aptitude is evident in any group of small children at play or in a dancing class. An analogy between speech and stance was drawn by Sheldon (1966): 'When a child has learnt to speak it takes further years to acquire a proper vocabulary; similarly it takes time to build up what one may term a vocabulary of posture—a collection of memories which will ensure an immediate and correct response to any and every deviation from the vertical.' Since these responses depend on the integrity of many interrelated neurological mechanisms, with final integration at cerebral cortical level, it is not surprising that performance deteriorates with ageing, and that deterioration is accelerated by the pathological changes of neurological or cerebrovascular diseases.

There are three attributes to consider:

1 *Posture:* alignment of the body segments properly in relation to one another
2 *Balance:* the ability to stand steadily
3 *Moving equipoise:* control of equilibrium in movement

Walking requires control of all three, and the neurological systems which provide it are:

1 *Muscle–joint sense.* Muscle spindle and tendon proprioception transmits essential information about length, tension, and speed of activity of muscle. This is monitored at higher levels:
   a brain stem: where reflex antigravity support is elicited through vestibulospinal and reticulospinal tracts in response to stretch stimuli
   b midbrain: where righting reflexes controlling posture and balance are elicited
   c cerebral cortex in the integration of patterned movements

2 *Basal ganglia.* These are concerned with posture other than antigravity support. They control postural integration of the body segments with each other and with equilibrium, at rest and in movement. This activity is complementary to antigravity mechanisms and they interact closely.

3 *Cerebellum.* This is concerned with reflex regulation of muscle contraction: with dynamic rather than static processes. It monitors the orders for movement issued by the cerebral cortex, compares what is happening with what should happen, and brings the force of muscle contraction into line with what is necessary.

4 *Cerebral cortex*. Here final integration of reflex and voluntary mechanisms occurs. It is often difficult to know how much is reflex and how much voluntary. Walking is usually thought to be voluntary, but the necessary actions are carried out perfectly with the mind entirely concentrated on other matters. It is at this level that failure of control of posture, of balance, or of equilibrium in movement must be compensated by conscious tricks and adaptations devised from experience and relearning. Unfortunately it is at this level also that evidence of depleted reserves often shows up first in old age, or in the pathological effects of cerebrovascular disease, so that defective postural control is not uncommon in old people, especially after strokes.

Balance exercises and constant practice are essential to encourage the best use of remaining compensatory mechanisms in a hemiplegic patient, but at best they can do no better than their peak level of attainment in earlier life. If a patient always walked like a cassowary before a stroke it is asking too much of rehabilitation to expect a walk like Margot Fonteyn's or Valery Panov's afterwards.

Difficulty in walking

Elderly patients often complain of difficulty in walking. The patient's, or the relative's, description of the difficulty must always be checked by personal observation of the gait, giving the patient space to walk freely and, if possible, to negotiate a few steps. This may be much more informative than neurological examination of old people who, frequently, have no ankle jerks, 'equivocal' plantar reflexes, no vibration sense, and show willing, but unhelpful, responses to other sensory testing.

Disorders of gait in old people fall into three groups: those often attributed simply to 'old age', which present without, or with indeterminate, clinical signs of neurological damage to explain the walking difficulty; those accompanied by signs of unilateral or bilateral corticospinal lesions; and those related to peripheral neuromuscular diseases.

Group A. Walking disorders often attributed to 'ageing' are:

1 A shortened step, walking on a wide base described as a *marche à petits pas* which may progress to shuffling with loss of arm swinging resembling parkinsonism.

2 Apractic disorders of gait where, in the absence of significant motor, sensory, or co-ordination deficits to account for loss of ability to walk, the patient seems unable to recall his former method of walking and although able to stand, and when supported, to lift each leg in turn over an obstruction such as a small stool or stick, cannot initiate a pattern of walking when left to himself, or, when started, to continue the movements for more than a few hesitant steps. Having come to a standstill, the hesitant movements can be started again only by coaxing and concentration for a limited period.

3 Loss of awareness of a true vertical stance. Some elderly patients, even after a brief illness, are unable to get up without help because they do not seem able to stand erect. When helped to get out of a chair they seem to thrust their body backwards instead of coming forward normally, and when they are pulled upright they lean 10 or 15° off-plumb backwards, or to one side or the other, and will fall unless supported. When asked to walk they will make appropriate leg movements of steppage, but they do not carry the trunk with them and appear to walk away from under their centre of gravity. It is as if the centre controlling vertical posture was set out of 'true'. It can be reset successfully in some patients by lying them on their faces for 15 or 20 minutes in bed, or on a tilting table, and by balance exercises in front of a long mirror so that the patient can see and help to make the necessary postural adjustments.

4 A reeling, unsteady gait punctuated by frequent falls may develop as a result of vertebral basilar insufficiency or other causes of degenerative changes in the brain stem and cerebellum.

Group B. There is evidence of focal corticospinal damage: spastic paresis of one or both legs, with altered reflexes and sensory or co-ordination deficits.

There are two critically important diagnoses to consider in this group. To miss either spells disaster for the patient.

1 *Spinal-cord tumour:* suggested by a slow onset of progressive weakness in the legs with diminishing range of activity, a history of preceding root pains, and a well-defined sensory level. Sphincter disturbance may be a late development. Possibilities vary from a neurofibroma (with *café-au-lait* spots and cutaneous neurofibromatosis) to malignant metastases or myelomatosis. A benign cord tumour is a neuro-surgical emergency because irreversible cord damage may develop quite rapidly and there should be no delay in seeking appropriate investigation.

2 *Subacute combined degeneration of the cord:* paraesthesiae in the feet, and later in the hands, often associated with intellectual decline, symmetrical spastic leg weakness, depressed knee and ankle jerks, extensor plantar reponses, and impaired joint-position and vibration sense in the legs. Early diagnosis (by investigation, of blood, bone marrow, vitamin B12 levels, and Schilling test) is essential because response to treatment is so good. (The neurological syndrome may anticipate the appearance of anaemia.)

Other causes of spastic paraparesis to consider are:

3 *Motor neuron disease:* an onset with symmetrical spastic leg weakness accompanied by fasciculation, wasting in the small muscles of the hands and in the shoulder girdle, and perhaps dysarthria. There are no sensory changes or sphincter disturbance.

4 *Cervical spondylosis:* perhaps a more common cause of leg weakness and unsteadiness in old age than is generally recognized. Onset is gradual with stiffness in both legs which are spastic on examination with increased reflexes, loss of vibration sense, and an ataxic gait with variable evidence of root involvement or dissociated sensory deficits. The most significant radiological change is narrowing of the spinal canal by posterior osteophytes in a lateral view (Matthews 1970).

5 *Prolapsed discs:* may mimic spinal cord tumour but are preceded usually by a long history of slowly progressive disability before paraplegia develops. At operation it may be possible to relieve pressure but more often than not the risks of attacking a calcified long-standing prolapsed disc are too great.

6 *Unknown causes of spastic paraplegia:* some will declare themselves in time: disseminated sclerosis, cervical spondylosis with myelopathy, chronic progressive cord dysfunction caused by vascular insufficiency, a parasaggital meningioma, and parkinsonism are possible causes of disordered gait where diagnosis may be uncertain or overlooked for some time.

7 *Ataxic gaits:* should perhaps be included here because so often they arise from a mixture of spasticity, weakness, sensory deficit, and a loss of balance involving disorders of cerebellar, spinal cord, and neuromuscular mechanisms. With cerebellar ataxia the patient *feels* and *is* unsteady, and has a waddling gait on a wide base and inability to walk steadily along a straight line or stand on one foot. 'Senile' or vascular or hereditary cerebellar degenerations, alcoholism, carcinomatous cerebellar neuropathy, myxoedema, or cerebellar tumours are amongst causes to investigate.

Group C. Disorders of gait related to deficits in sensory input, in peripheral nerves, and in muscles.

1 *Tabes dorsalis:* sensory ataxia causes the difficulty in walking. Lightening pains, Argyle Robertson pupils, incontinence with a large painless bladder, hypotonic legs with loss of reflexes and of deep pain sensation may be more useful indicators than tests of posterior column sensation or the Wassermann reaction. Tabes is rarely seen now.

2 *Peripheral weakness:* weakness and wasting of hip girdle and associated proximal antigravity supporting muscles may arise from neurological lesions:

    a cauda equina compression: N.B. 'saddle' anaesthesia
    b peripheral neuritis
    c acute polyneuritis
    d chronic peripheral neuropathy:

        i diabetes: usually with vascular disease (p. 67), patchy distal sensory changes; pain in calves, absent knee and ankle jerks, trophic changes in feet, autonomic changes (diarrhoea, incontinence, retention), often mild: *glucose-tolerance test*
        ii toxic: alcohol, sulphonamides, isoniazid, nitrofurantoin
        iii polyarteritis nodosa; paraesthesiae, weakness and palsies, raised erythrocyte sedimentation rate, electrophoretic pattern, eosinophilia
        iv sarcoidosis, reticuloses, carcinoma
    e myasthenia gravis
    f dystrophia myotonica: proximal leg weakness and falling, cataract: baldness, testicular atrophy, myotonic muscles
    g myopathy: hyperthyroidism, myxoedema, carcinoma, gastrectomy (osteomalacia and disordered calcium metabolism)

Faints

Old people use a variety of terms to describe transient disturbances of consciousness with, or without fits, e.g. an 'attack', 'weakness', a 'stroke', but neither these, nor the falls often associated with them, should be dismissed as a consequence of 'old age' without detailed inquiry about the nature of the attacks and appropriate investigation of them. A clear history may be difficult to elicit from a patient who is forgetful, or who loses consciousness without warning, and others who fall, especially those with drop attacks (p. 55), embarrassed by their inability to explain their frequent accidents, may be reluctant to volunteer information about them.

    The list of possible causes includes:

1 *Simple faints:* some old people are apt to faint with stress, heat, or pain, but as a new development investigation for anaemia or some other pathological state is necessary.
2 *Postural hypotension:* myocardial ischaemia or cerebrovascular insufficiency may cause dizziness or syncope on standing up too quickly, and some patients have persistent postural hypotension after strokes. Neither drugs nor elastic supports do much to help these patients and

if spontaneous improvement does not occur with time and increased well-being, as they recover, it is only possible to offer advice on taking precautions: to avoid very hot baths, dehydration (which would lower blood pressure), or strains which elicit the Valsalva manoeuvre (with chronic constipation).

3 *Carotid-sinus syndrome:* a hypersensitive carotid sinus is said to be a rare cause of vertigo, weakness, and convulsions in old people with hypertension, or with kinked atheromatous carotid arteries which are susceptible to pressure from a tight collar or forced head movements.

4 *Epilepsy:* idiopathic epilepsy, quiescent for some years, may reappear in old age but more commonly it is evidence of a newly acquired illness, perhaps the result of cerebrovascular disease or of a space-occupying lesion such as subdural haematoma, a cerebral tumour, or a metastasis. Transient confusion may be a post-epileptic phenomenon, following grand mal, petit mal, or jacksonian epileptic attacks. Myoclonic twitching or small involuntary movements may be early focal signs of a cerebral tumour.

5 *Stokes–Adams attacks:* caused by transient asystole with myocardial conduction defects. They are often so brief that some inactive old people are unaware of them, but in others who are up and about they are a source of very real distress because the victims are unable to protect themselves from the consequences of sudden loss of consciousness and falls which come on without warning. Repeated electrocardiogram tracings may fail to show satisfactory proof of abnormal cardiac rhythm, but every effort must be made to establish the diagnosis because a pacemaker can transform the patient's life as well as preserve it. Without this most of these patients fall victim sooner or later to fatal cardiac arrest.

Other causes of syncope to be excluded are covert painless cardiac infarction, supraventricular tachycardia, hypoglycaemia, vertebral basilar ischaemia, and adverse reaction to drugs—oversedation or idiosyncrasy may cause hypotension and vertigo, quite apart from toxic effects of poisoning with coal gas, alcohol, or other substances.

Falls

Interest in falls, as a leading cause of restricted activity, injury, premature breakdown, and even of unexpected deaths amongst old people, was first aroused by Sheldon (1948, 1960). He observed that:

1 women are far more liable to falls than men
2 the incidence of falls increases steadily with age in identical proportions for both sexes
3 falls are easily classified according to intrinsic or extrinsic causes

Underlying most falls there appears to be an age-related defect in the control of posture and gait. Sheldon (1966) devised a means of illustrating and measuring this, and attributed it partly to loss of neurons and biochemical changes in cerebellum, brain stem, and possibly other centres (see pp. 7–49) and partly to intermittent cerebral ischaemia—obstructive or hypotensive. These original findings have been confirmed in many other studies reviewed by Overstall (1978) but explanation of the 'senile decline in postural control' Sheldon described is still speculative, and it is still—apparently—irreversible.

Old people who fall may *trip* owing to senile, parkinsonian, ataxic, or apraxic disorders of gait; to impaired eyesight, visual inattention, or loss of concentration; or to lack of protection from extraneous domestic hazards such as ill-lighted steps, worn carpets, or loose wires; they may *stumble* because of clumsiness imposed by physical disabilities such as arthritis, the sequelae of injuries involving spine, pelvis, or legs, muscular weakness (osteomalacia; dystrophy), peripheral neuropathy, or covert pyramidal damage; they may *sway* owing to their deteriorating control of balance, or to vertigo caused by postural hypotension, adverse drug reaction (antihypertensives, diuretics, levadopa, phenothiazines, sedatives), or vertebral basilar insufficiency (cervical spondylosis, transient ischaemic attacks); they may *collapse* suddenly owing to cardiac syncope with loss of consciousness, or to drop attacks without loss of consciousness.

The limitations imposed on sensorimotor performance by ageing (Welford 1981) must add to the risk of falls from most of these causes, and may explain the increased incidence with age, and the sex differences, although this is more probably related to physical differences (which might include unsuitable shoes). Apart from altered sensory input from defective vision and labyrinths, weakened muscles, and stiffened joints, ageing impairs central perception, analysis, and integration in the brain, and reflex motor reaction in response to imbalance becomes slow and inaccurate (p. 50).

Drop attacks
Drop attacks are instantaneous falls, which occur almost exclusively in women, without warning, and without loss of consciousness (Sheldon 1948, 1963; Kremer 1958; Stevens and Mathews 1973). The patient may be moving about the house or out walking. Ability to stand upright is lost suddenly, the legs fold, and the victim 'falls in a heap', often with bruising, laceration, or more serious injury. The patient is often unable to get up unaided, but when helped up can usually stand and even walk, and may feel very foolish, being unable to account for the mishap. The immediate recovery of function once the patient is erect

was attributed, by Sheldon (1960), to the positive supporting reaction which revives lost tone in the antigravity muscles and restores normal higher centre control of posture and gait in response to pressure on the soles of the feet (the 'magnet response'), and Sheldon observed that it can be elicited in this way in patients prostrated after a drop attack as a means of helping them on to their feet.

Drop attacks are usually attributed to brain stem ischaemia, and the neurological deficit which may be responsible was discussed in detail by Kremer (1958). Compression or kinking of tortuous vertebral arteries owing to cervical spondylosis, or transient occlusion of small vessels by microemboli from atheromatous plaques, may explain some attacks. This theory is supported by the response sometimes obtained to anti-coagulants or drugs which suppress platelet stickiness. Anticoagulants may be considered too risky in old people, but anyone who is becoming incapacitated by the apprehension or the frequency of drop attacks deserves at least a 6–8 week trial of aspirin or sulphinypyrazone alone, or combined with dipyridamole.

The victims of falls usually recognize their failing but realize that there is little they can do about it other than to avoid sudden movement or changes of direction and protect themselves from environmental hazards which expose them to risk. They can be helped by imaginative advice on proper clothing (avoiding trailing garments or ill-fitting slippers) and on domestic aids (good lighting in passages and on stairs, uncluttered rooms, handrails, well-placed shelving and cupboards, and floors without loose mats or a high polish).

However, in an ageing population forgetfulness, apathy, and misfortune must continue to contribute to a rising incidence of falls. Moreover, Sheldon often quoted the comment from one of his patients 'once you are going, you have to go' to emphasize that the besetting weakness common to many old people who fall is their inability to regain balance once they lose it and begin to topple.

PARKINSONISM—LATE-ONSET DIABETES —ACCIDENTAL HYPOTHERMIA

These topics may seem incongruous in a section together, but they have at least four things in common:

1 peak incidence in the over-fifties
2 evidence of impaired autonomic nervous function
3 insidious onset, often missed
4 clinical picture often misleading; early diagnosis dependent on the serendipity of a good noticer (Asher 1960)

Parkinsonism

Paralysis agitans, the 'shaking palsy' described by James Parkinson in 1817, is one of the disorders comprising the parkinsonian syndrome characterized by tremor, muscular rigidity and slowing, weakness, and poverty of movement. References for details of the following outline are Calne (1970), Hornykiewicz (1975), Bianchine (1976), and Walton (1977).

Incidence and aetiology

Incidence in the general population of the United Kingdom is 1 in 1000, rising in the over-sixties to about 15 per 1000, and it presents in three main forms:

1 *Idiopathic parkinsonism:* paralysis agitans or Parkinson's disease
2 *Post-encephalic parkinsonism:* in survivors of the 1916–18 pandemic of encephalitis lethargica
3 *Symptomatic parkinsonism:* most common in older patients in association with:
  ● cerebrovascular disease
  ● phenothiazine intoxication

Rare aetiologies are head injury ('punch-drunk' elderly boxers); reserpine, carbon monoxide, or manganese toxicity; and other degenerative neurological disorders with parkinsonian features: syphilis, olivopontocerebellar degeneration, Behçet's disease, the parkinsonism–dementia picture of Jacob–Creutzfeldt disease or the Shy–Drager syndrome.

Most parkinsonism in elderly patients is either idiopathic or arteriopathic. A vascular aetiology is most likely when the onset is fairly sudden in late rather than middle life, with rigidity and bradykinesia more conspicuous than tremor, and with associated focal pyramidal damage, pseudobulbar palsy, and dementia, hypertension, or ischaemic heart disease.

Pathogenesis

The main pathological changes are extensive nerve cell destruction in the substantia nigra and globus pallidus, the appearance of spherical inclusions (Lewy bodies) in the nerve cells in these areas, and, in the later stages, a degree of cerebral atrophy and an excess of senile plaques and neurofibrillary tangles which may be out of keeping with the patient's age, and indicates a degenerative disorder extending beyond the basal ganglia (Hakim and Mathieson 1978).

The neurochemical deficiencies associated with parkinsonism were outlined in a concise review by Pearce (1978). Dopamine deficiency

(p. 61) is the most constant and most important of these, but anti-cholinergic drugs may enhance, or even better the response to dopamine replacement, implying that excessive cholinergic transmission is another factor in the underlying cause. It has been suggested that this stems from an increase in the cholinergic system brought about by a cholinergic takeover of the striatal receptors abandoned by failing dopaminergic neurons. There may be dopaminergic receptors, distinct from those affected in Parkinson's disease, involved in drug-induced and other dyskinesias, and neurotransmitters other than dopamine and acetylcholine, which also are depleted in parkinsonian brains, may contribute to the clinical picture: gamma aminobutyric acid (GABA) by releasing tremor and rigidity; serotonin by affecting motor behaviour through involuntary movements and myoclonus; noradrenalin, neural peptides, and monoamine oxidases by roles as yet undetermined.

Clinical picture
The symptoms and signs of parkinsonism are grouped under the following headings.

Appearance and attitude.
1 Unnatural immobility of facial muscles; impassive expression
2 wide palpebral fissures; diminished blinking and eye movements
3 slight or moderate flexion—head or shoulders, thorax, and pelvis
4 flexion and adduction of limbs at proximal joints
5 slight extension of wrists; fingers flexed at metacarpophalangeal joints and extended peripherally with thumb adducted and extended
6 equino-varus deformity of feet in late stages

Voluntary movement.
1 Slowness, more conspicuous than weakness, especially of small muscles, i.e. affecting eye movements (poor convergence), mastication, swallowing, articulation (monotonous slurred speech), and fine movements of fingers (writing, dressing, sewing, piano-playing)
2 associated and synergic movements impaired (arm-swinging in walking, gestures with speech)
3 paroxysms of akinesia (inability to initiate voluntary movement) complicate the variable state of bradykinesia (slowness of movements)

Muscular rigidity.
1 Agonists and antagonists uniformly affected, but distribution usually unequal on the two sides at onset
2 characteristically 'lead pipe' (plastic) unless tremor is evident when it becomes 'cog-wheel'
3 full range of movements can be elicited until contractures develop

Gait.
1 Akinesia may make it difficult to start walking
2 bradykinesia creates a shuffling walk of short steps which becomes 'festinant' when increasing flexion and diminishing control of equilibrium oblige the patient to catch up with his centre of gravity as it falls forward (or backwards)

Tremor.
1 Most conspicuous at rest
2 rhythmical, 4–6 per second
3 begins unilaterally, usually in an arm, and spreads to affect limbs and trunk, seldom the head
4 associated always with bradykinesia and extrapyramidal rigidity
5 increased by emotional upset
6 suppressed by voluntary movement, by conscious effort, and during sleep.

Autonomic disturbances.
1 Uncomfortable flushing, sweating, and seborrhoea
2 excessive salivation
3 toleration of cold better than of heat

Mental changes.
1 Irritability
2 depression
3 delirium
4 dementia

There is no sensory deficit, but most patients complain of crampy muscular pain, commonly attributed to 'rheumatism'. Inability to change posture without help often causes discomfort.

There are no reflex changes other than difficulty in eliciting tendon jerks as rigidity increases.

Course
Idiopathic parkinsonism follows a slow, unremitting course downhill towards total dependency and although modern treatment can remedy distress and discomfort and alleviate disability to some extent, it is only effective in bringing the patient back to an earlier, less impaired stage of the disease with symptomatic improvement; the underlying degeneration remains unchanged and the inexorable decline continues. Its rate is constant for the individual, but there are wide variations between individuals.

Dependency is the result of reduced range of activity, impaired control of posture, and loss of equilibrium with the constant risk of falls

leading to loss of confidence. In the advanced stages rigidity and contractures cause much discomfort and, perhaps, pressure sores. Mental
deterioration and incontinence often complete the picture of total
dependency. The time taken from onset to reach this stage is said to
be about twice the time from onset until the earliest evidence of dependency.

Diagnosis
Old people complain so often of slowing down, a sense of weakness,
tremor, or stiffness that it is only too easy to dismiss incipient parkinsonism as nothing more than 'old age'. Various other conditions with one
or more features resembling parkinsonism have to be considered in the
differential diagnosis, more especially since specific treatment with
levadopa was introduced.

Senile tremor.
1 Action tremor (induced and maintained by voluntary movement,
whereas parkinsonian tremor is static—maximal at rest)
2 finer and faster than parkinsonian tremor
3 affects the head most often (titubation), hands and fingers sometimes
4 no associated muscle weakness, slowness, or rigidity

Essential tremor.
1 Hereditary; onset in early life
2 action tremor of variable frequency
3 generalized distribution, *or* head, lips, and tongue only may be
affected
4 specific (temporary) relief with alcohol

Intention tremor.
1 Absent at rest, invoked by voluntary action, sometimes occurs with
precision movements in old age
2 associated with ataxia and other focal neurological signs in multiple
sclerosis or senile cerebellar atrophy

Dementia. Dementia is sometimes accompanied by variable rigid resistance to rapid passive movements (*gegenhalten*: 'holding against') and
by corresponding immobility, impaired postural control, and walking
apraxia. This may resemble parkinsonism but is distinguished from it
by the history of antecedent dementia, the absence of tremor, the nature
of the rigidity (as if the patient was actively suppressing attempted
passive movements), and by associated signs of arteriopathic dementia:

1 Generalized hyper-reflexia
2 positive snout and palmo-mental reflexes
3 pseudobulbar palsy

4 impaired postural fixation
5 tendency to fall backwards when standing

Biochemical basis of treatment
The complex interconnections of the basal ganglia are believed to
function, in the control of posture and movement, through the activity
of synaptic transmitters, particularly acetylcholine and dopamine. Most
of the dopamine in the normal brain is found in a tract which has been
defined between the substantia nigra and the caudate nucleus and
putamen. Cholinergic activity (excitatory) and dopaminergic (in-
hibitory) are normally held in balance in this nigrostriatal pathway.
Imbalance causes specific disorders of movement. For example dopamine overaction induces muscular hypotonia and the hyperkinetic
movements of Huntington's chorea or tardive dyskinesia, whereas deficiency produces the clinical features of Parkinson's disease.

Dopamine is a product of decarboxylation of its precursor levadopa.
Levadopa can cross the blood–brain barrier; dopamine cannot. The
simplified working hypothesis given above derives from research which
followed from experimental evidence in animals that levadopa could
reverse the effects of reserpine, and from the observation in psychiatric
wards that parkinsonism sometimes occurs as an adverse reaction to
treatment with reserpine. These basic data led to the discovery by
Hornykiewicz and his co-workers that levels of dopamine were grossly
depleted in the striatal brain tissues of patients who had died with
parkinsonism. Treatment with levadopa followed logically from this.

The cause of striatal dopamine deficiency underlying parkinsonism
is still unexplained, but degeneration in the nigrostriatal pathway is
accompanied by depletion of striatal dopamine which seems to follow
from primary degeneration in the substantia nigra. The brain can compensate for loss of dopamine for a long time (presumably by the biochemical activity of some still-active neurons) but deficiency eventually
exceeds the level of striatal compensation and symptoms appear.
Hornykiewicz suggests that the effect of treatment with levadopa is to
withdraw the patient from decompensation to a compensated state of
clinical parkinsonism.

Parkinsonism may be treated, therefore, by:

● drugs which enhance dopaminergic activity
● anticholinergic drugs
● mixtures of both

Idiopathic, post-encephalitic, and arteriosclerotic parkinsonism are
attributed to striatal dopamine deficiency and so may be expected to
respond to levadopa. Parkinsonism appearing as an adverse reaction

to phenothazines or reserpine is thought to occur because these drugs block transmission from the nigral cells to the dopamine receptors in the striatum. Dopamine output from the substantia nigra is actually increased to excess by striatal feedback without effect, so that treatment with levadopa is also ineffective, and anticholinergic drugs should be tried.

Drugs in parkinsonism
Cardinal principles in elderly patients (65+) are:

● small doses
● slow induction
● small increments at long intervals
● titration to individual need

Levadopa. Begin with 125 mg once or twice daily increasing by 125 mg increments twice weekly at most to a final level of 1·5–2·0 mg in six or eight weeks. About 75 per cent of patients respond, some extremely well, with early improvement in bradykinesia and rigidity. Tremor is slow to respond, if at all, and it may be many months before full benefit is gained in better posture and muscle strength, lessened sialorrhoea and sebum secretion, and even improved mental capacity.

Reserpine, phenothiazines, and monoamine oxidase inhibitors should not be prescribed for patients on levadopa. Pyridoxine affects the metabolism of levadopa and may reduce its side-effects (but of course it may also impair the efficacy of levadopa therapy if vitamin preparations containing pyridoxine are given at the same time).

Carbidopa, a decarboxylase inhibitor which does not pass the blood–brain barrier, was introduced to reduce decarboxylation of levadopa in peripheral tissues and so enable more to reach the striatum without increasing the dose. Sinamet contains 0·25 mg carbidopa and 250 mg levadopa, or 10 mg carbidopa and 100 mg levadopa (Sinamet-110). Slow induction with the smaller dose is appropriate in geriatric practice. If levadopa is already being given it should be omitted for 12 hours before giving Sinamet, and the initial dose should be about one-quarter of the previous dose of levadopa.

The advantages claimed for combined therapy are a quicker therapeutic response (in days instead of weeks); less nausea and vomiting; the 'on–off' phenomenon is less in evidence; the daily dose of levadopa can be much increased without the risk of adverse reactions; and that cardiac arrhythmias are less troublesome.

Complications and adverse reactions: from a six-year review of levadopa therapy, Shaw *et al.* (1980) conclude that it improves the quality of life and, probably, life expectancy for most patients who can tolerate the drug for more than two years, but there is a substantial failure rate.

Early failure may result from inadequate response or from *side-effects*:

1 *Psychiatric* (see below)

2 *Gastro-intestinal* (anorexia, nausea, vomiting): reduce the dose; give levadopa *with* food; do *not* give phenothiazine anti-emetics

3 *Cardiovascular* (postural hypotension, arrhythmias): may be controlled with propranolol

Late failure usually follows either from waning of the benefit obtained from each dose with early morning akinesia and increasing disability ('wearing-off effect'). or from intolerable *adverse reactions*:

1 *Involuntary movements:* mild dyskinesias may appear within the first two years of treatment, becoming more severe and generalized, as orofacial dyskinesia, cramps and dystonic deformity of limbs, nocturnal myoclonus, or rocking and twisting movements of head, trunk, or limbs.

2 *Psychiatric disorders:* commonly necessitate stopping levadopa treatment. Toxic confusion may develop at any stage; visual hallucinations may appear with increasing intensity as treatment continues; dementia is a distressing complication in 25–30 per cent of patients; paranoid delusions and depression also occur.

3 *On–off phenomenon:* unaccountable and unpredictable swings from activity to immobility develop in some patients. There may be several changes within the hour, of alarming severity with sweating, flushing, palpitations, and a rise in blood pressure as mobility returns. They may represent variations in the plasma level of levadopa and their severity is reduced by lowering the dose.

Bromocriptine. Bromocriptine, a dopamine agonist, thought at first to be an alternative to levadopa, has limited uses. It is less effective than levadopa and is equally liable to cause adverse reactions. It may be tried alone in mild parkinsonism to defer introducing levadopa for a year or two, but its best use is to supplement conventional Sinamet therapy which has had to be reduced owing to side-effects or waning response. Worthwhile clinical improvement, more even therapeutic effect, and control of on–off phenomena or dyskinesia may be obtained more successfully with the mixture than with either drug alone (Pearce and Pearce 1978).

Bromocriptine is supplied in 2·5 mg and 10 mg tablets, and 5–10 mg is about equivalent to 100 mg levadopa combined with carbidopa. Careful titration of treatment is essential as with levadopa, beginning with 2·5 mg after the evening meal, increased only by 2·5 mg twice each week until response is satisfactory, usually around 40 mg daily in divided doses. Further increases if necessary may be made with 10 mg tablets at six- or eight-hour intervals.

Anticholinergics. These are largely replaced by levadopa, but many patients still derive benefit from them, alone or in combination with levadopa. The most popular drugs are:

- benzhexol (Artane) 1–10 mg
- benztropine mesylate (Cogentin) 0·5–6 mg
- procyclidine hydrochlor (Kemedrin) 1–10 mg
- orphenadrine hydrochlor (Disipal) 50–300 mg

All may improve tremor, rigidity, and bradykinesia and dry up sialorrhoea. Older patients are especially at risk of side-effects including blurred vision, agitation and hallucinations, confusion, and retention (a special risk in old men with prostatic dysuria).

Amantadine hydrochlor (Symmetrel). This drug (50–200 mg) is thought to release dopamine from intact dopaminergic terminals in the nigro-striatum, and its effect is enhanced by levadopa given with it. However, in elderly patients its benefits are apt to be outweighed by its adverse reactions, the most conspicuous being agitated restlessness, nightmares, hallucinations, and mental confusion.

General management
Old people do not show the dramatic response sometimes obtained with levadopa at the onset of paralysis agitans in middle-aged patients. Even when there is marked improvement in rigidity and bradykinesia the elderly patient may still be handicapped heavily by loss of normal postural fixation, unpractised righting reflexes, the weakness of disused muscles, and loss of confidence and of incentive. The loosening up and improved morale gained from a successful response to levadopa must be used to best advantage in a systematic programme of rehabilitation. Grant (1963) and Hurwitz (1964) described the aids and techniques required from physiotherapist and occupational therapist in combined courses of treatment. The patient with parkinsonism will need them, either as out-patient or in-patient, at intervals determined by individual need, for the rest of active life, to prevent relapse into abnormal postures and immobility. They comprise:

1 *Postural and balance exercises before a mirror* (parkinsonian patients are often unaware of abnormal posture or changes in position and need visual clues to make corrections).

2 *Practice in turning in bed; chair drill* (perhaps with a raised seat).

3 *Walking exercise:* steppage is unimpaired in parkinsonism, and walking can be encouraged, even in patients who cannot sit or stand properly, provided they are supported from behind by a hand in each axilla and rocked gently from side to side in time to shift weight to each leg in turn as it moves forward. Aids to walking are raised heels or a weighted jacket for patients who tend to fall backwards, and lines painted on the floor, or coloured tiles, 18 inches apart, to encourage rhythmical, even steps.

4 *Dressing, bathing, and toilet practice:* in parkinsonism associated with arteriosclerosis the instance of dementia is high and mental deterioration limits the possibilities of re-education owing to impaired grasp, concentration, and memory.

5 *Routine nursing:*
  a frequent changes of position to prevent discomfort and bedsores
  b an air- or water-filled mattress and chair seat
  c prepared food and perhaps help with feeding (especially to ensure enough fluid intake to avoid dehydration)
  d aperients or enemata to prevent constipation and impaction causing spurious diarrhoea
  e special attention to bathing and hygiene of contracted limbs

Insomnia may be relieved by *diphenhydramine* (50 mg) which has a mild anticholinergic action, and *imipramine* (10–30 mg) may be required for depression. Above all the patient and relatives need unfailing support and encouragement from the family doctor.

Late-onset diabetes

Age and obesity are the outstanding factors predisposing to diabetes mellitus and most diabetics, when first diagnosed, are well over 50 years old (the age of peak incidence). Epidemiological studies from Bedford (Sharp *et al.* 1964) and elsewhere have shown that:

1 Blood glucose levels rise or glucose tolerance declines with age.
2 The incidence of diabetes increases with each decade, especially over 50 years of age.
3 There are wide individual variations in renal glucose threshold and these too are age-related. It is low in youth and high in the elderly so that false *positive* glycosuria is common in the young and false *negative* in the old (Butterfield *et al.* 1967; Jarrett 1976).
4 Glycosuria therefore is not a reliable screening test for diabetes, and estimates of blood glucose are necessary to pick up lesser degrees of glucose intolerance.

5 Screening by this means indicates that there is at least as much un-known diabetes in the community as is known to exist, especially amongst people who are old and fat.
6 It may be difficult to decide how to interpret borderline abnormality in glucose tolerance and when to treat asymptomatic diabetes. Where there is doubt, long-term follow up is necessary because frank diabetes develops in later years in many instances, and there is a high risk of complications, especially blindness.

Clinical picture

The clinical picture of diabetes and its onset are different in old age than in youth. Juvenile diabetes is usually an acute illness and the classical symptoms—thirst, polyuria, wasting, and ketoacidosis—are severe, leading rapidly to prostration and coma if untreated. The cause is hyperglycaemia owing to insulin deficiency, the renal glucose thres-hold is exceeded creating an osmotic diuresis, and impaired glucose and ketone metabolism lead to metabolic acidosis and alterations in acid–base and water balance. With increasing dehydration, peripheral circulatory failure and reduced glomerular filtration add to the hyper-glycaemia. Hyperosmolarity then aggravates the intracellular de-hydration and combines with ketoacidosis to cause drowsiness, acidotic 'air hunger', and eventual coma.

The onset of diabetes in old age is sometimes as sudden and severe as in youth but more often it is gradual and less dramatic. Hyper-glycaemia is the result of inactivation of insulin or impaired tissue re-sponse to it, rather than from insulin deficiency. A raised renal glucose threshold may limit glycosuria and osmotic diuresis, even with a high level of blood glucose. Metabolic acidosis is slower to develop, but is frequently fatal, being unrecognized for what it is.

Late-onset diabetes, therefore, is more often detected as a result of a urine test in routine medical examination, for insurance perhaps; or owing to mild symptoms such as pruritis, paraesthesiac, or unaccount-able nocturnal diarrhoea; or because investigation is made necessary by one of the major complications. These are described in the next section.

Complications

Coma. Three varieties occur in late-onset diabetes:

1 *Diabetic crisis:* the hyperglycaemic ketoacidosis described earlier. Mortality in the elderly is high because diabetes has not been diagnosed early enough or owing to the seriousness of an illness which has caused the deterioration; for example, a hidden infection in chest, genito-urinary system or abdomen, or a vascular thrombosis.

2 *Hypoglycaemic coma:* a serious risk to elderly diabetics. Inaccuracies in self-administration of antidiabetic therapy, cumulative effects of chlorpropamide, or potentiation of oral antidiabetic drugs are the most likely causes (p. 70).

3 *Hyperosmolar non-ketoacidotic coma:* some mild late-onset diabetics seem able to cope with their defective glucose metabolism, even when it deteriorates, without resorting to fat as a source of energy, and so they may become extremely hyperglycaemic without developing ketosis. Some, admitted in impending coma, have had blood glucose levels of 48–60 mmol/l (8–10 g/l) or more. Serum sodium and urea are raised, with intense haemoconcentration and hyperosmolarity but no keto-acidosis. As in diabetic crisis coma probably follows from hyperosmolar intracellular dehydration, and mortality is high unless the diagnosis is made in time to correct this with appropriate parenteral infusions and insulin dosage determined by frequent assessment of the clinical state and the blood biochemistry of the patient. Early indications of this complication may be a capricious desire for sweets or sugary soft drinks accompanied by weakness, thirst, and polyuria which may be disregarded or attributed to a diuretic as drowsiness and confusion lead on to coma.

Ocular complications. The risk of blindness in the late-onset diabetic is ten times greater than the risk to a non-diabetic from all other causes (Caird *et al.* 1969). *Diabetic retinopathy*, the most important cause, begins with capillary aneurysms and retinal venous varicosities in the macular area, progressing to white, waxy exudates and thromboses or 'blot' haemorrhages causing ischaemia or detachment. *Diabetic cataract* resembles other senile varieties but appears 10 or 15 years earlier.

Vascular disease. There is much uncertainty about the relationship between the metabolic abnormalities of diabetes and the pathogenesis of atheroma. However, diabetics develop atheroma earlier and more extensively than non-diabetics and are at greatly increased risk of ischaemic heart disease, cerebrovascular accidents, and peripheral vascular occlusions with gangrene. Hyperglycaemia is only one of many factors linked with atheromatosis of larger vessels, but it is accepted as the primary cause of the microvascular degeneration underlying diabetic retinopathy and the glomerulosclerosis which leads to hypertension and renal failure as diabetic complications.

Diabetic polyneuritis. Diabetic polyneuritis is a demyelinating neuropathy of uncertain pathogenesis, possibly the result of vascular degeneration involving the vasa nervorum. The legs are most affected with either

1 pure sensory neuropathy causing burning paraesthesiae (especially at night), pain in the calves, and sensory ataxia owing to loss of postural sensibility or
2 mixed patterns of neuropathy with muscular weakness and diminished tendon reflexes as well as sensory symptoms

Complications attributed to impaired autonomic nervous function are:

- pupillary abnormalities
- disordered sweating
- altered gut motility (constipation or nocturnal diarrhoea)
- loss of bladder tone: impotence
- postural hypotension.

Diabetic foot. Diabetics are predisposed to trophic changes in bone and soft tissues, and to gangrene of toes and feet, owing to neuropathy and ischaemia. Meticulous preventive measures are essential: regular chiropody, well-fitting shoes, advice on foot care, and immediate attention to any signs of abrasion or infection.

Management
Elderly diabetics are said to divide about equally into three groups: those whose hyperglycaemia can be controlled on diet alone; those who need insulin; and those who respond to antidiabetic drugs. Each group presents its own problems.

Diet. Weight reduction by restriction of calories and carbohydrate is essential for the overweight patient and may control hyperglycaemia even in those who are not. Some weeks of strict dieting may be necessary before results show, and reducing diets often fail in geriatric practice. Sometimes the patient cannot understand or remember the simplest rules, and others cannot or will not comply with them owing to confusion or to the feckless attitude expressed in remarks such as 'I've had my diet—I'm having my dinner now'. Protein is an expensive alternative to carbohydrate and elaborate diets are a nuisance at any time, not least for relatives who are responsible for preparing food and for seeing that the patient does not overeat.

Insulin. Patients who need insulin are those with:

- classical onset when thin and underweight
- ketoacidosis
- complications and associated illness, especially infection
- inadequate control with trial of diet and hypoglycaemic drugs.

Daily injections may be tolerated as a necessary evil by the old ager, but failing vision, loss of dexterity, and shrinking from self-administration are difficulties that make special demands on relatives or on nursing services.

Antidiabetic drugs. Oral hypoglycaemic agents have solved difficulties for a large number of late-onset diabetics. Tolbutamide and chlorpropamide are still widely used and although the 'second generation' sulphonylureas have not been shown to have significant long-term advantages they are now being increasingly prescribed (e.g.: Glibenclamide).

The sulphonylureas act only in patients still able to produce some endogenous insulin, which explains their special value in late-onset diabetes. They promote insulin release from the β-islet cells and probably enhance its peripheral activity. Side-effects occur more often with chlorpropamide and although they are few, some are serious, but occur seldom:

- allergic skin reactions
- sensitivity to alcohol: flushing and dizziness
- blood dyscrasias
- jaundice

Hypoglycaemia is a risk with both drugs, but more so with chlorpropamide which is cumulative. Secondary failure (loss of its effect), occurs within two years in a proportion of patients treated with tolbutamide.

The *biguanides* phenformin and metaformin were once recommended for very obese patients who showed no response to determined efforts to reduce weight by diet, or to supplement tolbutamide if secondary failure should occur. However, the action of these drugs in diabetes is not known; they are more toxic than sulphonylureas, causing gastrointestinal upsets in almost half of the patients treated; and lactic acidosis may be a fatal complication of treatment with phenformin in patients with hypoxic illnesses, alcoholism, and liver or renal failure. The patient who needs phenformin will probably need insulin sooner or later.

Apart from these immediate side-effects, the long-term safety of oral antidiabetic drugs has been questioned, and their use has been modified in the United States, following a report from the University Group Diabetes Program showing a significantly higher frequency of deaths from cardiovascular disease in tolbutamide-treated patients. Further long-term studies are required (Jarrett 1976), and meanwhile the well-tried value of sulphonylureas should not be denied to those elderly diabetics whose risks of reduced life-expectancy from cardiovascular causes may be far outweighed by the risks of blindness, and for whom oral antidiabetic therapy may be much more convenient and appropriate than insulin.

Drug interactions
Finally, because old people are so often the victims of polypharmacy, the late-onset diabetic is at special risk of certain drug interactions causing unexpected changes in blood glucose concentration.

Increased blood glucose. Thiazide diuretics, phenatoin, and corticosteroids impair insulin secretion. Oestrogens, thyroid drugs, levadopa, and morphine exacerbate diabetes.

Decreased blood glucose. Sulphonamides, salicylates, and phenylbutazone displace sulphonylureas from protein-binding sites and so enhance their effects. Barbiturates, mono-amine oxidase inhibitors, and propranolol lower blood glucose levels and enhance the effect of sulphonylureas.

Accidental hypothermia

Hypothermia is defined as a central body temperature below 35 °C (95 °F). 'Accidental' hypothermia, occurring fortuitously, is distinguished from low temperatures induced as part of medical or surgical treatment.

In Great Britain accidental hypothermia—'being old in the cold' (*British Medical Journal* 1977)—has been recognized for many years as a special hazard of old age. Surveys have indicated that many old people are at risk in the winter because their body temperatures and the room-temperatures of their homes are too low; that some thousands of old people admitted to our hospitals each winter are hypothermic; and that considerable numbers die, or make chance recoveries, from unrecognized accidental hypothermia.

There is a steady output of body heat from metabolic activity. More heat is generated in response to cooling by *muscular activity* (voluntary exercise or involuntary shivering) and by *cutaneous vasoconstriction* which reduces heat loss from exposed areas of skin, and enhances the thermal insulation of subcutaneous fat and layers of clothing. This is the most important defence mechanism against cold and without it temperature continues to drop in spite of shivering.

Regulation of body heat is monitored by the hypothalamus through the autonomic nervous system. Like other homeostatic mechanisms responsible for the constancy of the *milieu intérieur* its efficiency and responsiveness are apt to be impaired by age changes. The more important limitations are *diminished sensory input* (so that an old person may be unaware of being cold), *absence of shivering* (as an indicator of falling temperature), and *defective vasoconstriction* (as a protective response to cold). Illnesses leading to physical handicap and mental incompetence may further limit capacity to generate and maintain body heat. The *endogenous causes* of hypothermia (Exton-Smith *et al.* 1964) are:

1 Those relating to sheer *old age*:
   a impaired temperature regulation
   b infirmity and immobility
   c slowness
2 *Malnutrition* (lowering metabolic activity and stamina)
3 *Illness*:
   a endocrine (myxoedema; hypopituitarism)
   b neurological (falls; drop attacks; strokes; head injury; parkinsonism; paraplegia)
   c mental deterioration (slowing up and lack of awareness)
   d circulatory collapse (infarction; haemorrhage; infections)
4 *Reaction to drugs*:
   a sedation (reduced activity; drowsiness; coma)
   b vasodilation and diminished shivering (alcohol, phenothiazines, sedatives, and anti-depressants have all been incriminated)

The *exogenous cause* (or precipitating factor) is exposure to cold, self-inflicted by a parsimonious ageing recluse or an eccentric fresh-air fiend, or inadvertent, but inevitable, in a frail social isolate without the clothing, bedding, fuel, or food to maintain body heat. In these conditions some old people succumb without even an illness or accident to account for hypothermia, but there are others whose intrinsic ability to generate and maintain their own body heat is so severely impaired that they become hypothermic even when tucked up and apparently well-insulated against the cold in a hospital bed.

Symptoms and signs
As body temperature drops towards hypothermic levels greyish pallor and facial puffiness develop, suggestive of the cold skin and lethargy of myxoedema. There is muscular rigidity, slowing of pulse and respirations, the blood pressure falls, and the patient becomes apathetic and drowsy. Below 32 °C (90 °F) confusion progresses to coma. Delayed intraventricular conduction and heart block with a characteristic 'J' wave (an extra upward deflection at the junction of QRS and ST segments) or atrial fibrillation appear in the electrocardiogram in many patients. The deep, frigid cold to be sensed on palpation of the viscera below the rigid abdominal wall is a measure of the low core temperature. In the extreme stage complications include broncho-

pneumonia, vascular thromboses (cardiac infarct), haemorrhages, gangrene, pancreatitis, and visceral necroses.

Prevention
Mortality is high because hypothermia itself is dangerous and because underlying disorders are often serious. *Prevention* is better than cure.

1 *Anticipation* through surveillance of old people at risk (p. 27).
2 *Clothing and bedding* designed to prevent heat loss, especially from head and extremities: dispose of out-worn matted woollens and supply mittens, knitted cap, bedsocks, long underwear, and warm dry blankets (lightweight 'space' blankets may become available).
3 *Safe heating appliances:* electric *over*-blanket (the under-blanket is too dangerous if incontinence occurs); effective *roof insulation*; *double glazing*; easily accessible *power points for supplementary heating*.
4 Enough *food* at all times and extra food in winter ('warmth' from alcohol is an illusion: it increases heat loss from the body).
5 Encourage as much *activity* as possible. Not even polar clothing can prevent a normal person in a cold room from losing heat if he remains sedentary (*British Medical Journal* 1977).
6 Check *core body temperature* of suspects. Use a low-reading thermometer (either rectal reading or temperature of a urine specimen collected in a bottle specially designed to record it (Fox *et al.* 1971)).

Treatment
If domestic circumstances permit it may be possible to rewarm a patient with a mild degree of hypothermia at home, with extra blankets and room temperature raised to 22–27 °C, but an intra-rectal temperature approaching 35 °C or less demands emergency admission to hospital to monitor progress and forestall complications. Continuous supervision is necessary to strike the balance between the dangers of collapse owing to rewarming too fast, or of irreversible tissue damage when it is too slow. Essentials in treatment are:

Moderate hypothermia (35–32 °C).

1 Barrier-nurse in a single cubicle with special precautions against pressure sores.
2 Handle gently and with as little demand on effort from the patient as possible to avoid precipitating ventricular fibrillation.
3 Record rectal temperature, pulse, respiration, and blood pressure hourly.
4 Insulate with woollen blankets against further heat loss.
5 Raise room temperature to 27°C to bring the patients deep body

temperature up at about 0·5 °C every hour. If not rising fast enough raise the room temperature to 28–32 °C; if rising too fast a fall in blood pressure may indicate an urgent need to cool the room and the patient temporarily.

6 Analyse arterial blood gas and acid–base regularly; and estimates of blood glucose concentration may be indicated.

7 Oxygen may be needed for anoxia, and fluids and sodium bicarbonate to combat dehydration and metabolic acidosis.

8 An antibiotic (such as ampicillin) should be given whether bronchopneumonia has been diagnosed or not.

Severe hypothermia (32 °C or less). Additional needs are:

1 Admission to an intensive care unit.

2 Oxygen by endotracheal tube with intermittent positive pressure ventilation.

3 Arterial and venous catheters for blood sampling, pressure monitoring, warmed intravenous fluids, and control of metabolic acidosis.

4 Hydrocortisone 100 mg 6-hourly has been recommended but it is doubtful whether it (or any other drug) will help if the patient is unable to respond to these practical measures.

CONSTIPATION—INCONTINENCE—PRESSURE SORES

Constipation

Constipation is a common complaint in geriatric patients. Not as many are constipated as believe they are (Agate 1972), but it often contributes to discomfort, restlessness, and incontinence; and an advanced state of faecal impaction is a potentially lethal condition (Anderson 1971).

Chyme passing from ileum to colon changes to formed faecal mass by withdrawal of water and salts through the bowel wall. Transit times are 3–6 hours in the small intestine followed by 36–72 hours in the colon; 5 days is the accepted upper limit of normal. An ageing colon can work within this for old people who are active, but considerable delays in transit times have been demonstrated in sedentary old-agers and chronic invalids (Brocklehurst 1973), and it is quite normal to expect wide individual variations (from several times daily to less than once a week) in the frequency of rectal emptying. The normal impulse to defaecate is a response to a mass peristaltic movement of the colon propelling the faecal mass into the rectum, and it may be initiated and reinforced by increased intra-abdominal pressure involving posture and contraction of abdominal muscles, voluntary or involuntary.

Factors which promote constipation involve:

1 Patient's way of life (often associated with mental deterioration):
   a lack of roughage, fruit, and vegetables in diet
   b dehydration
   c inactivity (especially confinement to bed)
   d neglect of the normal impulse resulting in eventual suppression
   e persistent misuse of laxatives
2 Age changes (factors causing muscular weakness):
   a age changes in abdominal and pelvic muscles
   b diminished intestinal reflex
      i age changes in colon musculature
      ii loss of mucosal sensitivity
   c obesity and sedentary habits
   d abdominal distention (idiopathic megacolon; volvulus)
   e multiple pregnancies
3 Illness:
   a debilitating illnesses
   b causes of local pain (fissure; haemorrhoids)
   c depression
   d paraplegia and other neurological diseases
   e hypothyroidism

Treatment is as much a medical as a nursing responsibility and entails explanation and discussion, general measures (diet, regular habits, exercise); adjustment of fluid intake (especially early in the day) and choice of a suitable laxative. (Refer for details to Agate (1972) and to Brocklehurst (1973).)

Incontinence

Incontinence, as a personal disorder, has been defined as 'loss of urine at any time except when desired by the individual' (Yeates 1976). In old age, however, the definition must cover degrees varying from occasional stress 'accidents' to persistent inability to contain urine or faeces, night and day, recognized or unrecognized by the patient; and it must distinguish also between incontinence which is a misfortune of involuntary loss of control, or of inappropriate, but voluntary, voiding as a feature of psychiatric illness.

Want of agreement in definitions explains discrepancies in estimates of prevalence of incontinence, but it is thought that in the United Kingdom the rate may be 20 per cent or more amongst people aged 65+ in the community, and that it may vary from 25 to 50 per cent in patients under geriatric medical or psychiatric care in hospital (Willington 1976).

Incontinence is a symptom, not a disease, and there are multiple factors associated with it. The outstanding single cause of intractable difficulties is the development of an uninhibited neurogenic bladder associated with intellectual deterioration, disorientation, and signs of degenerative or vascular brain damage.

Normal micturition requires control at three levels in the nervous system:

1 The sacral reflex arc (S2, 3, and 4), through sympathetic and para-sympathetic innervation maintains bladder 'tone' in a state of small continuous, intrinsic, detrusor contractions. In response to bladder filling (i.e. stretch) it summates them into more forceful isolated contractions, relaxes the sphincter, and initiates emptying.
2 The midbrain centre is probably concerned in reflex inhibition or reinforcement of the micturition reflex.
3 The frontal cortex, where voluntary control of inhibition or excitation develops in early childhood.

As the bladder fills, tension is monitored at higher levels and detrusor contraction is inhibited until the owner becomes aware of the rising tension when the information is relayed to the cortex. Then micturition is either deferred by conscious inhibition, or initiated by voluntary detrusor contraction and sphincter relaxation when time and place are appropriate. Lesions in this system at different levels produce four types of neurogenic bladder:

1 The autonomous bladder: cauda equina lesions disrupt afferent and efferent innervation causing irregular, inefficient reflex emptying.
2 The atonic neurogenic bladder: in tabes or peripheral neuropathy, with lesions of posterior nerve roots, the disruption of the afferent component causes retention with overflow from an insensitive over-distended bladder.
3 The reflex neurogenic bladder: in spinal-cord lesions the sacral arc is intact but, when deprived of control from higher levels, an insensitive incontinent paraplegic bladder empties reflexly at frequent intervals.
4 The uninhibited neurogenic bladder: results from general or focal brain damage involving frontal cortex. Deprived of normal voluntary control a spastic contracted bladder develops, with incontinent emptying in response to low filling levels, the pattern so often associated with ageing, mental deterioration, and cerebrovascular accidents.

Assessment of the incontinent patient
Continence is amongst the body mechanisms impaired in old age by poverty of reserves, and management of failure to maintain it is best

considered in terms of *predisposing* and *precipitating* factors (Brocklehurst 1951).

Conditions which predispose to incontinence are:

1 A hyperexcitable neurogenic bladder owing to deteriorating cortical inhibition, which probably occurs more often than is generally appreciated.
2 Anatomical aberrations at the bladder neck, a commonplace in old age, especially amongst elderly women.
3 Idiopathic histological age changes in genito-urinary tissues may be another contributory factor.

Legions of old people adapt to increasing precipitancy and dysuria, devising ways and means to stay dry within the limits imposed by their physical and mental agility and the convenience of their domestic arrangements. However, for many of them, the balance between these eventually becomes so unstable that even a minor illness, injury, or change in social circumstances is enough to upset it and to destroy the ability to cope with a badly functioning bladder. Precipitating factors which bring this about may be considered as *intrinsic* (those within the patient), or *extrinsic* (those relating to his environment).

Intrinsic factors include:

1 The progressive immobility of arthritis, parkinsonism, and other causes of unsteadiness and difficulty in walking (pp. 48–56), which may be made worse suddenly by an illness or a fall, extinguishing the last remnants of fading independence.
2 Local irritation owing to cystitis and other genito-urinary infections; cystic calculi; polypi; urethral caruncle; faecal impaction.
3 Clouded consciousness from any cause (p. 35) often precipitates incontinence, transient perhaps, resolving with recovery from the underlying illness, but too often persisting as a latent dementia may persist once uncovered by an extraneous upset imposed on poverty of reserves p. 9).

Extrinsic factors are:

1 Inaccessible or inconvenient toilet facilities (chairs too low; bed too high; no handrails on passageways, steps, or bathroom; lavatory out-of-doors; no commode available at night).
2 A combination of social isolation, physical handicap, and not enough help.
3 A move to strange surroundings (e.g. hospital).
4 Unimaginative routine management designed more for nursing convenience than for consideration of the individual and anticipation of need.

5 Premature assumption that incontinence is inevitable, applying a negative routine of 'mopping up' tactics instead of positive remedial measures.

Faecal incontinence
Most victims of this complaint are in long-stay geriatric or psychiatric wards, and their incontinence is often the reason for admission. Brocklehurst describes three main causes:

1 Local diseases causing intractable diarrhoea:
  - colitis; diverticulitis
  - carcinoma of colon or rectum
  - diabetic neuropathy
  - drug idiosyncrasy
2 Faecal impaction with chronic constipation.
3 Neurogenic changes allied to those causing urinary incontinence.

Treatment
Some years ago Newman (1962) observed that it was no good looking for information on incontinence in the textbooks because they were 'written by people who do not have any problem with it'. This is not true of the textbooks of geriatric medicine which have appeared since then with well-informed sections on incontinence derived from research, much of it initiated by geriatric physicians. The most recent is a treatise edited by Willington (1976) compiling expert opinion on every aspect of incontinence in old age—medical, surgical, gynaecological, psychiatric, nursing, and sociological. These textbooks should be consulted for details of equipment and methods. Only some general principles are given here.

The day-to-day care of an incontinent patient is carried, inevitably, by relatives and nurses, but the attending doctor's assessment and informed opinion are essential to the design of an effective plan of treatment.

It has been well said that there is 'an unconditional need for kindness in its treatment'. There is no excuse for inconsiderate behaviour or open rudeness to incontinent patients, and senior staff, both doctors and nurses, have an obligation to ensure, by constant vigilance, that untrained staff and relatives understand and act upon this. The following difficulties, common to most elderly incontinent invalids, should be explained:

1 the lack of awareness of those with clouded consciousness
2 the frequent impairment of sensory perception
3 difficulties of communication with deaf or dysphasic patients

4 self-consciousness of those with insight and concern (especially women), and the postural difficulties endured by many of them who have to contend with arthritis and other deformities when trying to use a bed-pan
5 the restlessness and confusion often caused by retention
6 mishaps caused by inability to handle bottles
7 the effects of over-sedation and potent diuretics
8 the aggravation caused by apprehension, anxiety, and neglect of efficient routine management

The assessment outlined earlier may be used to distinguish three groups of patients as a guide to treatment:

Group 1. Those who are mentally clear, aware of their mishaps, distressed by them, and willing to co-operate in efforts to regain control. Some may be helped to become more mobile and so to stay dry (e.g. with levadopa in parkinsonism that has been overlooked; with imipramine in depression; or by a spring-loaded seat for an arthritic cripple who cannot get out of his chair). Cystometry may help others (Wilson 1948, 1976). Yet others may respond to close supervision and insistence on well-timed visits to the toilet, to the guidance and aids of an occupational therapy department or, when all else fails, to the special garments, appliances, and protective techniques advised by Willington (1976).

Group 2. Patients who are mentally clouded (in the delirium of acute illness, after injury, or in post-operative recovery). If control of continence was reliable before they became ill, they may be expected to recover it if the illness responds to treatment, but those who have brain damage, especially from head injury or stroke, may need protracted treatment under a positive, well-planned programme to give them their best chance of recovery. The essentials are these:

1 to have the patient up and about as much as possible to discourage drowsy apathy and bedsores (N.B. care with sedatives)
2 regular visits to the toilet, two- or three-hourly, and careful skin cleansing with soap and water followed by a protective cream.
3 limited fluid intake after 6 p.m. *but* give adequate fluids *early* in the day
4 make sure that constipation is not contributing to incontinence
5 keep a chart to assess the patient's needs, as a guide to progress, and as a stimulus to a systematic and meticulous nursing routine
6 explain progress to the patient who can understand it and reward success by sympathy and encouragement
7 try cystometry to assess the state of the bladder musculature and, if it is uninhibited and hyperactive, as a means of 'increasing control of

the voiding reflex and improving the capacity of the bladder' (Wilson 1976).

Group 3. This is the group with *intractable incontinence* beyond the patient's own control, occasionally for a physical reason (such as an inoperable neoplasm with a fistula), but more often because of dementia. For these patients well-planned 'management' attaining the best possible standards of care is the aim rather than 'treatment' implying hopes of a cure. There are relatively few of these invalids in the geriatric population as a whole, but together the problems of domestic, nursing, and medical care they represent are disproportionately heavy. Incontinence is often the last straw that breaks willingness of a family to continue looking after an aged invalid, and it is quoted as a prominent cause of admission for long-stay institutional care. Both in the home, where the family need maximum support, and in hospitals and nursing homes where it is equally important to the nursing staff, everything possible should be done:

1 to make sure that no patient whose incontinence *might* respond to treatment escapes the net of thorough assessment; and
2 to see that everything that might be done *is* done to minimize the burden of care of those whose incontinence must persist. The routines and resources for this set out by Willington include:
  a nursing practice and communication with the patient
  b monitoring by electronic 'dampness detectors'
  c special devices—urinals, collecting bags, hygienic pants/pads/clothing
  d design and use of catheters

As the number of confused incontinent long-stay patients increases so does the risk of accumulating large concentrates of them in hospitals and nursing homes. The burden of time-consuming bathing, cleansing, changing, and sorting of foul linen may then outweigh other aspects of nursing care and defeat the best efforts of senior staff to uphold good standards and morale. It would seem that modern hospital authorities have an obligation to devise some system of equitable distribution of small manageable groups of these long-stay patients amongst the clinical departments in units designed to provide maximum nursing convenience. They should have:

1 the most up-to-date labour saving equipment for bathing, lifting and handling heavily disabled elderly invalids
2 constant access to modern methods of foul-linen disposal (and this is essential to the proper management of such invalids at home)
3 an unfailing flow of the supplies (linen, clothing, pads, dressings,

barrier creams, and other comforts) essential to ensure hygienic methods of incontinence management

4 the advice and support of doctors interested in the control of infection, restlessness, discomfort, nutritional, and other problems of long-stay and terminal care

Given these resources, and with enough staff directed by informed senior nurses, it should be possible to do away with the more repellant features and the unspoken resentment associated with this aspect of geriatric nursing.

Bedsores and the treatment of pressure points

The myths and old wives' tales relating to the prevention and treatment of bedsores were described some years ago by Bliss, McLaren, and Exton-Smith (1966). 'Infallible' methods recommended in the past include: fortification of patients with extra proteins, vitamins, anabolic hormones, insulin and antibiotics; skin protection with ether, alcohol, soap, silicone, creams, sticking plaster, or photographer's rubber cement; treatment of sores with chlorophyll, brine, sugar, enzymes, jam, vitamin E, dried plasma, honey, antibiotics, tannic acid, oxygen, Marmite, ultraviolet light, sunlight, electric light, plastic sprays, or the juice of a South American plant *Santella asiatica*; plastic operations— either removing slough or leaving it; appliances such as plastic beds, air beds, water beds, sawdust beds, sheepskins, mats of rubber spikes, sorbo foam or plastic foam; and finally, patients have been massaged, ventilated, strapped in machines which turn them over, tipped from side to side, supported on points under them, immersed in water, suspended in hammocks or by wires passed through the iliac crests and clavicles; three even had their bony prominences excised.

Good results were claimed for all these methods, but no controlled trials were done until Bliss and her colleagues carried out theirs to investigate the value of the alternating-pressure mattress. They concluded that whilst standard intelligent nursing practice is enough to prevent pressure sores amongst a few patients at risk, it is inadequate to cope with the needs of large concentrates of heavily disabled aged sick.

There are two types of bedsore: superficial and deep.

Superficial abrasions. Some thin, ageing skins are more susceptible to injury than others, and vulnerability is greater when the patient is thin, malnourished, on steroid therapy, or when the skin is macerated by incontinence or affected by skin disease or drug rashes. Restlessness, or failure to lift the patient properly when changing sheets, may be enough to produce superficial abrasions which are extremely painful and add to the patient's distress. Pain is reduced and healing occurs quickly if the lesion is kept clean with careful skin toilet, covered with a non-stick dressing (tulle-gras), kept dry, and free from infection and from further pressure. If so, changing at most every second day will allow epithelium to grow, but restlessness and incontinence delay the process, and dry dressings or too frequent changes strip off the newly proliferated healing tissues.

These superficial lesions are preventable, and their appearance reflects shortcomings in patient care—perhaps lack of vigilance, staff shortage, mishandling of a heavy patient, defective control of incontinence, or inadequate sedation.

Deep ('malignant') pressure sores. These are true 'pressure' sores, and predisposing factors are:

1 lowered tissue vitality in debilitating illnesses
2 impaired peripheral circulation in hypotensive states
3 sensory and motor deficits which keep a patient from moving or realizing the need to do so

Under these conditions local thrombosis of vessels may occur in the deep tissues overlying bony prominences, even with pressures which normally would have no ill effects. Duration of pressure is more important than its intensity (heavier patients are usually better cushioned against their own obesity), so prolonged immobility is the real danger—in lengthy operations under anaesthesia, after strokes, in parkinsonism, or in the comatose lethargy with low blood pressure following cardiac infarction, internal haemorrhage, or over-sedation.

The patient may not complain, or may be too ill to notice discomfort, and the first evidence of the sore is brawny reddening of the skin appearing within 24 hours, but necrosis will have begun already in deeper tissues, including muscle. The next stage is superficial blistering which breaks down in a day or two exposing full-thickness skin damage with a necrotic central slough indicating the deeper necrosis extending to bone. The slough, which often becomes black, does not separate spontaneously for many weeks. Secondary infection develops in fascial layers, undercutting the surrounding skin. Cellulitis and pocketing, sometimes with anaerobes, creates a resistant focus of infection which erodes debilitated defence mechanisms. At best a bedsore delays recovery, sometimes for months. At worst it is the fatal last straw.

Prevention
There is no better evidence in medicine than a bedsore that 'prevention is better than cure'. Susceptibility is determined by *general condition,*

mental state, physical capacity, and *incontinence.* The risk is greatest in the first ten days after onset of illness or admission to hospital. Doctors and nurses should recognize the onset of apathy, loss of appetite, and incontinence as early signs of deterioration, and shiny reddening, blistering, or induration of the skin as evidence of incipient breakdown. Unremitting special nursing may have to be continued for weeks until the patient's skin condition is consistently good, and all signs of pressure effects have disappeared. It involves:

1 constant changes of position—turning 2-hourly or even half-hourly when at high risk: sitting out of bed when fit to do so (but unfit patients may then be liable to develop pressure sores over ischial tuberosities and heels).
2 care with sedatives to compromise between traumatic restlessness and stuporose immobility.
3 correction of the effects of malnutrition: hypoproteinaemia, anaemia, and vitamin deficiency.
4 avoiding dehydration and maintaining blood pressure and cardiac output, if necessary by intravenous infusions or transfusion.
5 use of an alternating-pressure air bed or water bed in the 'high-risk' period or with precarious patients. Special beds have been shown to reduce the incidence of bedsores but they are *not* substitutes for traditional good nursing practice. This still recognizes the development of a bedsore as an admission of failure (Agate 1972).

Treatment
If breakdown occurs preventive measures should be reviewed and reinforced if necessary to make good fluid and protein loss (from serous or purulent discharge), to provide the means of repair (vitamin supplements), to combat general infections (pneumonia; cystitis), and to remedy the anaemia anticipated in any chronic infective condition.

The essentials of local treatment are:

1 cleaning and dressing a painful infected lesion with its penetrating sinuses
2 identification and eradication of specific local infections, and prevention of re-infection
3 promotion of granulation and encouragement of healing

Daily irrigation with warm saline, or with saline and peroxide mixed half-and-half, helps to wash out debris and pus, to reduce anaerobic organisms, to encourage separation of slough, and to limit the pocketing of infection in deeper tissues.

Healing cannot begin until the slough separates. Spontaneous debridgement is very slow in large pressure sores, but surgical intervention has to be selective because some patients are unfit for it. If so, hot packs of hypertonic sodium sulphate solution, of 1/2000 Eusol, or of strepto-kinase and streptodornase may encourage separation of slough and keep the patient comfortable. The packs must be big enough to cover the area, and must not be allowed to dry, and so stick to painful abraded tissues. Dressings are best held in place by large binders or elastic tubular-mesh bandages. It may be necessary to catheterize an in-continent patient, to protect the dressing but this should be discontinued as soon as possible. When the general condition is improving and granulation gives evidence of healing, excision and grafting may be considered.

MALNUTRITION—MALABSORPTION— METABOLIC BONE DISEASE

Malnutrition

Old age leads to physical and mental infirmity, social isolation, or deprivation of one kind and another to such an extent that malnutrition might be expected to occur often amongst old people in their homes. Indeed, the incidence of clinical or subclinical nutritional deficiency in elderly patients admitted to hospital is quite high, but it is also quite misleading. The evidence from surveys in Great Britain, and the United States (Agate 1972, Brocklehurst 1973) support the finding originally made by Sheldon (1948), that the general nutritional state of the overwhelming majority of old people in their homes was normal, or at least as good as his own, even under stringent post-war rationing. In both Sheldon's survey, and those more recently carried out for the Department of Health and Social Security in the United Kingdom, only 3 per cent of the old people visited were considered to be mal-nourished. The cause, often self-evident, was usually to be found in prolonged illness, in disabilities leading to limited mobility, in mental disorder, or in domestic difficulties. Malnutrition is usually the conse-quence, not the cause, of disorders such as dementia or depression, or occasionally of the personality disorder known as the Diogenes Syn-drome (Clark *et al.*, 1975). This unusual condition occurs in people who, although often well-educated and of good family background, with-draw from society, cut themselves off from friends and relatives, rejecting help of any kind, and live in squalid isolation in some attic, basement cellar, or outhouse until admission to hospital is forced on them owing to weakness and inability to resist. They are apathetic, but not dementing, refuse to discuss their motives, and their deprivation is evident in their state of filth and infestation as well as starvation.

Advanced signs of malnutrition are listlessness, hypothermia, pallor, pinched facies with sunken eyes, slow pulse, low blood pressure, and oedema. This develops when osmotic changes caused by negative nitrogen balance and hypoproteinaemia combine with water and salt retention brought about by renal insufficiency and by altered adrenal corticoid activity.

It is easy to recognize florid malnutrition such as this, with signs of avitaminosis, but it is rare, and it is difficult to prevent, because to reach such levels of deprivation often means that it has been intentional. The more common and preventable borderline or subclinical nutritional deficiencies of old people are sometimes more difficult to identify and have to be anticipated by applying a good index of suspicion to old people 'at risk' (p. 27). Besides great age, infirmity, multiple pathology, and dietary indiscretion, living alone, depression, bereavement, poor housing, and distance from shops contribute to isolation and loss of interest in preparing a sufficiently varied diet. Malnutrition such as this must underlie or add to much ill-health in many old people. It is difficult to estimate how much or how many, because so far surveys and research have not revealed what are the precise nutritional needs of old people. Therefore there is no definition of what constitutes under-nutrition or over-nutrition for an ageing individual.

Food intake must be related to the output of energy, and most people do eat less as they get older and less active, although a few, especially older women, become overweight because they persist with a calorie intake more appropriate to their expenditure of energy 10 or 20 years earlier. The problem is to ensure that old people can afford, and will take the trouble, to acquire and to prepare food of the quality they need to keep fit. Prescribed diets are no use. Better to encourage freedom of choice and the fun of experimenting with soups and cooking varied menus. Advise not too little, but not too much, ringing the changes in food, as they can afford it, from the different groups:

1 dairy foods: cheese and eggs; red meats; poultry and fish
2 wholemeal bread; cereals, preferably those with high bran content
3 fresh vegetables; salads, as much as they can afford and will eat; fresh fruit
4 at least 3 pints of fluid intake daily (including 1 pint of milk)

Advise elderly people to have a good and varied diet and to cultivate the habit of systematic preparation of good food. They should avoid insidious short-changing 'with tea and biscuits'. Simple cooking methods are advisable, for which the old-ager will need a convenient little oven, a good fridge, a food blender, and disposable aluminium foil.

There is no means of knowing whether the vitamin intake amounts to the desirable levels and if there is doubt it is wise, and will certainly do no harm, to add a multivite tablet daily for one month in three. Estimated daily needs are 5000 i.u. vitamin A, 0·8 mg B_1, 1·3 mg B_2, 1·0 mg B_{12}, 250 μg folic acid, 50 mg vitamin C, and 250 i.u. vitamin D.

Vitamin A deficiency is probably rare, but subclinical B_1 deficiency possibly contributes to congestive heart failure in some patients; paraesthesiae, cramps, weak and tender calf muscles, and a Korsakow state of memory impairment are evidences of B_1 deficiency, or even a risk of Wernicke's ophthalmoplegia, especially if protracted intravenous feeding is given without vitamin supplements. Evidence of thiamin deficiency has been found amongst long-stay hospital patients. Angular stomatitis and atrophic changes in the mucosae of mouth and tongue, diarrhoea, and mental changes may indicate ariboflavinosis or nicotinic-acid deficiencies (provided oral abnormalities are not attributable to dentures, drug idiosyncrasy, or deficiency of iron). Folic-acid levels are frequently low in old people, not necessarily with associated anaemia, and the incidence of atrophic gastritis and pernicious anaemia both rise with age, and with a corresponding fall in serum B_{12}.

The clinical evidences of ascorbic acid deficiency are fatigue, hyperkeratosis of hair follicles with curled hairs (especially on the abdomen), perifollicular haemorrhages, petechiae around feet and ankles, 'sheet' haemorrhages, subcuticular ecchymoses over the thighs, and sometimes more extensive intramuscular or intra-articular bleeding. Edentulous patients do not develop gingivitis. Delayed healing of infected operation scars or bedsores may be the result of frank vitamin C deficiency or of an increased demand for tissue repair which exceeds a marginal reserve.

Vitamin D deficiency is discussed under metabolic bone disease.

The best treatment of malnutrition is intelligent anticipation. Advice on diet is properly included in pre-retirement courses, and it should be a special feature of the preventive care of 'at risk' old-agers. Food intake will have to be limited to milk, purées, and supplements until a severely malnourished patient can tolerate more solid diet.

Malabsorption

Malabsorption was once known as steatorrhoea because this, and the diarrhoea associated with it, were the most obvious features, but the entire clinical picture includes malnutrition and the signs of defective absorption of other nutrients:

1 weight loss, sore tongue, and lassitude
2 loose bulky motions with a high fat content (steatorrhoea is excretion greater than 6 g daily on a mixed diet containing at least 50 g of fat)
3 anaemia (iron, folic acid, and B_{12} deficiencies)
4 haemorrhagic tendency (hypoprothrombinaemia)
5 cramps and tetany (low serum Ca and P)
6 osteomalacia (lack of vitamin D)
7 epithelial changes and neuropathy (other vitamin deficiencies).

The source of malabsorption in old people may be found in:

1 stomach: partial gastrectomy; pernicious anaemia
2 digestion: biliary or pancreatic deficiencies
3 small intestine: resection; blind loops and fistulae; coeliac disease (gluten enteropathy)
4 vascular occlusion: intestinal angina (superior mesenteric artery)

Partial gastrectomy is one of the more common causes of the malabsorption syndrome, and patients who survive into old age with their partial gastrectomies are especially prone to develop osteomalacia. However, it has been shown that vitamin D absorption in post-gastrectomy osteomalacia is impaired very slightly, if at all, and it seems more likely that the association of osteomalacia with partial gastrectomy in the elderly is the result of a dietary vitamin D deficiency, not malabsorption.

The incidence of malabsorption in old age is probably much higher than is appreciated. Diarrhoea is uncommon, and lassitude, weakness, and weight loss are insidious symptoms often attributed simply to ageing. Old people may fail to appreciate the significance of long-standing flatulence and altered bowel habit, and have to be asked direct questions about frequent or abnormal stools. Malabsorption is often diagnosed as a result of investigations to account for a refractory megaloblastic anaemia. They should include:

● 3-day stool specimens for fat analysis
● serum carotene
● full blood count and bone marrow
● glucose-tolerance test
● xylose excretion
● plasma proteins and electrophoresis
● serum vitamin B_{12} and Schilling test
● electrolytes (especially Ca, P, and alkaline phosphatase)
● X-ray chest and pelvis
● gastrointestinal barium studies
● jejunal biopsy?

The last of these should not be imposed lightly on a frail or confused old person when the results of therapeutic trial of a gluten-free diet, folic acid 15 mg by mouth daily, vitamin B_{12} 100 μg intramuscularly weekly, and iron if necessary, may be most effective within a few weeks.

Metabolic bone disease

Old people present most often with *osteoporosis*: bone loss from an otherwise normal skeleton; less commonly with *osteomalacia*: deficient calcification of normal bone osteoid. Both conditions are generalized, affecting the whole skeleton, unlike *Paget's disease*, a disorder of un-known aetiology with successive osteolytic and osteoblastic activity affecting areas of the skeleton with patchy asymmetry.

OSTEOPOROSIS

Bone loss occurs with ageing, corresponding to atrophic age changes in other tissues and, as in these, the distinction between 'physiological' age-related osteoporosis and 'pathological' osteoporosis is difficult to define.

Bone development and bone loss have been assessed from radio-graphs by estimates of bone density, and by indices derived from measurement of bone thickness (isotope-absorption techniques are now being devised). Studies have shown that bone mass increases rapidly in childhood and adolescence until the individual is fully grown. The increase continues less rapidly until middle life, when bone loss begins. The skeletal prospects of each individual, therefore, are determined to some extent by the quantity, or the quality, of the bone they have acquired at this point, quite apart from the rate or the extent of sub-sequent bone loss. Everyone loses bone as they grow older, and average loss is the same regardless of how much they begin with, so that in old age osteoporosis may follow what would be accepted as normal bone loss from a skeleton which, at best, only reached a relatively low level of mineral content. Factors which influence the bone mass attained at maturity are sex (girls develop less than boys), race, nutrition, physical activity, endocrine function, and illness.

Bone loss, beginning at about 45 years of age, progresses most rapidly in women for about 10 years after the menopause, continuing into late life, contrasting with men, whose bone loss begins to diminish entering their seventies, and who even show some increase in their eighties. This appears to correspond with the survival into extreme old age of an élitist group of exceptional old people who retain good health and vigour. Sheldon observed that this applies more to men than to women, and perhaps these very special old men have better than average skeletons too. About 25 per cent of women aged 65 and over are osteoporotic to the extent of increased liability to fractures compared with about 5 per cent of men. By 70 years of age many elderly women have lost half of their peak levels of bone development.

Bone loss with age follows various patterns:

1 Slow loss: normal bone ageing, onset 40–5 years, predominantly in post-menopausal woman
2 Rapid loss: both sexes, at any age in adult life. These acute exacerbations of bone loss are unexplained, although hormonal imbalance, nutritional factors, or the restricted activity of disabling illnesses are suspect

Specific causes
● immobility (sedentary life, fractures, strokes)
● corticosteroid excess (Cushing's disease, steroid therapy)
● alcoholism (dietary deficiencies)
● rheumatoid arthritis (unrelated to cortico-steroid therapy)
● hypogonadism
● nutritional factors (protein, calcium, fluoride, and vitamin deficiencies)

Diagnosis
Suspect osteoporosis in the elderly patient with signs of collapse of vertebral bodies, i.e.:

● kyphosis ('dowager's hump')
● diminished distance between head and symphysis (crown–pubis should equal pubis–heel)
● a redundant fold of abdominal skin
● pain in the back radiating around the trunk or to the legs
● lower ribs overriding iliac crests

There are three diagnostic X-ray features: ghost-like appearance of bones; biconcave shape of vertebrae; and small proportions of compact to cancellous bone in shafts of long bones. Serum calcium, phosphate, and alkaline phosphatase are normal. Diagnosis depends on exclusion of other bone diseases and abnormal blood chemistry. Osteoporosis is sometimes accompanied by osteomalacia which may contribute to it.

Treatment
This is prolonged: reassurance is important. Post-menopausal bone loss may be reduced if oestrogen therapy is started within three years of the menopause—Tab. Premarin (conjugated oestrogens 0·625 mg) one daily for 21 days followed by 7 days without. This cycle could be con-

tinued for a year or 18 months, but it does not follow that the bone loss is a sequel of oestrogen deficiency alone. It is at least as important to limit the two factors most likely to increase bone loss: bed rest and steroid therapy.

Treatment of established osteoporosis includes:

1 high calcium diet (plenty of milk, 2–4 g calcium lactate or gluconate daily)
2 anabolic steroid—nandrolene decanoate, two courses at intervals of 6 months of a single intramuscular injection of 100 mg at intervals of 3 weeks and lasting 12 weeks
3 activity
4 spinal support, if tolerated
5 calciferol if alkaline phosphatase is raised

Difficulties arise because the interplay of underlying factors is not fully understood, because all age-related changes will correlate with bone mineral loss, and because osteoporosis tends to improve spontaneously with few vertebral fractures, less pain, and a slower or arrested height loss. Hence *every* advocated treatment may appear to give improvement regardless of the method of assessment.

OSTEOMALACIA

Osteomalacia is a disease caused by lack of vitamin D, now recognized to be, or to act in its hydroxylated form, as a hormone. Its precursors in the skin (dehydrocholesterol) and food (ergosterol) can be converted by sunlight into vitamin D (calciferol) which is inert until hydroxylated, first by liver enzymes into 25-hydroxycholecalciferol (25-HCC) and then in the kidney to 1,25-dihydroxycholecalciferol (1,25-DHCC) which mediates both calcium absorption from the gut and its mobilization from bone by specific action on skeletal osteoid. The synthesis of 1,25-DHCC may be controlled by the parathyroid gland in response to serum levels of calcium or factors responsive to them.

Osteomalacia is not uncommon. The incidence is high in women over 70 years of age, living alone, house-bound and malnourished, and as a late complication of partial gastrectomy or other causes of malabsorption. Lack of sunshine may be as important a contributory factor as nutritional deficiency.

In old people osteomalacia is easily overlooked. It may be confused or may co-exist with osteoporosis. Besides the indications already mentioned the diagnostic index of suspicion includes:

● vague generalized aches and pains
● low backache
● muscle weakness and stiffness

- waddling gait (proximal muscle weakness)
- skeletal deformities
- bone pain and tenderness

X-rays show bone rarefaction, and occasionally there are pseudo-fractures (Looser zones) in the pubic rami, femoral neck or shaft, axillary border of the scapula, ribs, or upper end of humerus.

Investigations include:

- serum proteins, which affects serum Ca and P levels
- blood urea, which affects serum Ca and P levels
- 24-hour urinary Ca excretion
- serum Ca: should be low or normal
- serum P: should be low
- alkaline phosphatase: should be raised
- faecal fat
- blood count; erythrocyte sedimentation rate
- ? bone biopsy (iliac crest), often the only means of confirming the diagnosis (wide uncalcified osteoid seams).

Treatment

Prophylaxis. In housebound elderly women, 10–20 μg vitamin D daily. Tablet of calcium with vitamin D (500 i.u.) or vitamin A and D capsules (450 i.u.) 1 daily for 3–4 winter months. Encourage exposure to sunlight.

Therapeutic. Begin with 50 000 i.u. of vitamin D (1·25 mg calciferol) daily for two weeks, or until relief from pain is obtained. Then reduce to a maintenance dose of 10 000 i.u. daily or 2 tablets of calcium and vitamin D (1000 i.u.) daily for 12 months, with winter prophylaxis to follow. It may be wise to assume that there is coincidental osteoporosis and give a high calcium intake and anabolic steroids as well.

PAGET'S DISEASE

Paget's disease is not regarded as metabolic bone disease but if its osteolytic phase predominates it may occasionally mimic osteoporosis. Its aetiology is unknown, and its incidence increases in frequency after middle life to affect about 10 per cent of the population aged 90 and over. Bones affected in order of frequency are pelvis, femur, skull, tibia, lumbo-sacral spine, dorsal spine, clavicles, and ribs.

The characteristic pathophysiology is increased bone resorption accompanied by increased bone formation in a pattern of imbalanced phases of activity and inactivity. In active phases resorption predominates in bones which are brittle, soft, and highly vascular. As this osteolytic activity decreases the bone becomes less vascular and new dense, hard bone is formed. In the active phases serum alkaline phosphatase levels may be exceptionally high. Serum calcium and phosphorus are usually normal.

Clinical evidence of Paget's disease is variable. The disease may only be discovered in a routine X-ray for some other reason, or may present with progressive deformities and pressure effects. Bone pains, headache, eighth nerve deafness, brain-stem or spinal cord compression with paraplegia and high-output heart failure are possible complications. The prospects for some patients have been transformed since calcitonin, injected once or twice daily, has been shown to relieve bone pain and alleviate compression effects such as deafness or incipient paraplegia.

TERMINAL CARE—SEDATION—CONTROL OF PAIN

Terminal care

Attitudes to fatal illness have changed in the second half of this century.

1 It has become possible to prolong existence on a scale unknown to former generations, owing to progress in medicine and methods of resuscitation and intensive care. This has raised ethical problems of prolonged dying which were equally unknown.
2 Mortality rates were once so high, especially in infancy and adolescence, that death was accepted with a philosophical resignation that is less evident today, even in reactions to the deaths of very old people. Death in early life evokes concern, not passive acceptance, and it has become more difficult to decide when heroic efforts to maintain life should give way to the measures necessary to provide only comfort and freedom from anxiety.
3 This dilemma causes more heart-searching in the care of children and young adults than of elderly invalids, but it should not be supposed that because old people are reticent and withdrawn they are any less anxious or worried about their illnesses, or their prospects. Today the greatest misfortune facing the patient who is not going to get better is the danger of being neglected, not in clinical attention from nurses and doctors, but in being denied time to talk, to ask questions, and to escape from a feeling of being isolated, set apart as someone who is not participating properly in the 'recovery game'.
4 There are so many stimulants, sedatives, and analgesics available that it has become increasingly difficult to decide what is best to pre-

scribe to control anxiety, pain or depression. All doctors and nurses involved in clinical practice need to have some special knowledge of the
range of drugs to choose from and the limitations, as well as the scope of
their therapeutic effects.

5 It used to be thought that few people approaching death realized
that it was the probable outcome of their illness, or gave much thought
to it. Lord Horder, 35 years ago, wrote that realization of impending
death was 'rare'. Recent studies, on the contrary, have shown that
three out of four patients with inoperable cancer are well aware of what
was about to happen to them, and that many old people in their last
weeks, although perhaps not realizing how close the sands are to running out, do consider the possibility, spend a lot of time thinking about
it, and may wish someone would offer to discuss it with them. Few
people worry about being dead; it is the prospect of what they may
have to face in the process of dying that is the usual source of anxiety
in those who ask about it, and they need reassurance most about relief
of pain, of breathlessness, or of a sense of suffocation.

6 There is a need for more accommodation to provide terminal care
as a special service, not only for old agers, but for all those with fatal
illnesses who cannot be looked after properly at home. It can be argued
that money would be better spent extending domestic services to ensure
that everyone can end their days in comfort in their own homes, but
often this is not the best arrangement for all concerned. Belief that
everyone should die at home is like belief in euthanasia; those who are
its strongest supporters are usually those who believe that 'it is something that is very good for other people' (Anderson 1973). Young
families in overcrowded dwellings, or a household of dependent ancients, however willing, cannot be expected to cope with the exacting
problems of heavy or prolonged terminal nursing and to contrive the
proper standards of care. (The reasons for the growing load of dependency and the shortfall in resources to deal with it are discussed on
pp. 20, 21, and 23.)

Terminal care begins when it has been decided that there is nothing
to gain from efforts to prolong survival and that the aim of further
treatment should be to 'ease the passing'. Dr. Cicely Saunders (1963)
defined this as the stage when 'definitive treatment gives way to symptomatic treatment'. The decision to make the change rests with the
doctor, whose clinical judgement must answer the question: 'is the illness terminal?' It is an important decision, because of its influence on
treatment and on the attitudes of all who attend the patient. It is also
a difficult decision because if the patient is to be treated as if he were
dying, it must be known that he *is* dying, and, even if the diagnosis

is accurate, old people have a perverse way of recovering unexpectedly, and contrary to even an experienced medical opinion.

Saunders (1978) edited a series of essays which represent the collective wisdom and experience of colleagues engaged with her over many years in the day to day care of the dying and in the research she initiated on the management of terminal illness in St. Christopher's hospice.

Management
The essentials in management are these:

1 The patient must be assured of basic comforts warmth, fluids, food, and friends. Incontinence is an embarrassment to patients who still retain consciousness and normal insight, and are distressed by a physical liability they cannot themselves avoid imposing on others. Every effort should be made to deal with it for them.
2 Persistent pyrexial illness, with diminished fluid and food intake, predispose to dehydration, chronic constipation, faecal impaction, and intolerable discomfort. Responsibility for assessment and treatment is as much medical as nursing. A routine ward blue-print of treatment is no substitute for the individual consideration each patient needs, including, quite often, relief of local pain from fissure or haemorrhoids.
3 Electrolyte imbalance may result in the apathy and asthenia of salt or potassium depletion. It is also important to make sure that protracted intravenous fluids are accompanied by an appropriate intake of vitamins. If intravenous dextrose is given over long periods without thiamin a Wernicke–Korsakow ophthalmoplegic confusional state may be superimposed on clouded consciousness. Reference has been made earlier (p. 85) to the need for ascorbic acid and vitamins A and D.
4 Effective communication between patient, nurses, doctor, and relatives must be assured. The patient should be given time, if the wish seems to be there, to talk about his anxieties.
5 Consideration should be given to necessary support for those about to be bereaved. A determined effort should be made to anticipate and to prevent subsequent isolation of the bereaved member of an elderly couple. Otherwise the survivor may become completely cut off and devastated by the loss of a spouse. Neglect of ordinary interests and of diet may quickly reduce them to a state of apathy and rapid deterioration. In domestic practice it is important to arrange pre-bereavement and post-bereavement visiting of the elderly by nurses or social workers who are best able to anticipate what the outcome of the death of one of an elderly couple may be. This is worthwhile preventive medical care. Domiciliary services should be notified of all instances of terminal illness where the caring relatives are old people, and there should be good

liaison between the hospital service and the community health team.

6 Communication calls for special comment. It is often asked: 'what should the patient with terminal cancer be told?' but it is wiser to ask the question: 'What do you let your patient tell you?' The patient should be given every opportunity to talk without being pushed into an unwanted discussion. They need a good listener, not an inquisitor. 'Listening itself can be the therapeutic' (Saunders). The doctor who thinks patients know only what he tells them deludes himself. Discerning patients take in much more than we give them credit for, from the behaviour of the staff, from our attitudes on ward rounds, and from the events they are involved in (visits to the X-ray department, investigations, or visits to other hospital units). Fear of loneliness and isolation, or depression and resentment of dependence on nursing staff and others, increase apprehension and add to problems they can resolve only by freedom to talk about them. Sympathetic and informed listening from someone able to bridge the communication gap helps to reduce family anxiety and constraint. A doctor, himself the victim of an incurable illness, said that as a dying patient all he felt that he could do for his family was to keep them from realizing how much he minded the prospect. Fortunately, most patients, like him, are 'strong in courage and in commonsense'.

To sum up:

1 do not thrust information on the patient
2 avoid empty reassurances or deliberate prevarication
3 when a patient wants to talk decide who is best able to meet their need—doctor, medical social worker, nurse, or chaplain
4 see that companionship is assured; avoid isolation
5 create a sense of security and confidence by the verbal assurance that pain and anxiety *can and will* be controlled

Finally, there are the disturbances of mental function sometimes amounting to what Saunders defined as 'mental pain'. About one-third of dying patients become confused, either as a result of their illness, or perhaps because of the drugs they are given to relieve their symptoms. This clouded consciousness can make things easier for them, and for their relatives. In others, however, evidence of mental distress may arise from the combination of anxiety and dyspnoea; a sense of constant breathlessness, of impending suffocation, may be frightening and unbearable. The depression of terminal illness may be intensified if there is constant nausea and sickness, or even more so if there is a sense of guilt or self-consciousness provoked by persistent incontinence (as we have seen earlier), or perhaps by the necessity to deal with offensive dressings. These anxieties, like other mental torment, may be harder to relieve than physical pain.

Sedation

The following notes refer to geriatric sedation in general as well as in terminal illness.

Sedatives and tranquillizers should not be prescribed for old people until every effort has been made to find out why a patient is sleepless or restless, and to resolve causes of anxiety, deprivation, or discomfort (p. 36). A change of position, a hot drink, and a few kind words are often more effective than medicine. Indeed, far from controlling confused restlessness, some sedatives increase it.

As always, accurate diagnosis is the only basis for treatment. It is no use giving hypnotics or tranquillizers to relieve insomnia caused by pain (often vague and unidentified in old age). Nor is it necessary to give powerful analgesics to settle a bewildered old invalid disorientated by a move into hospital, or an old man who has always had a nightcap of whisky and still needs it.

When drugs have to be prescribed it is best to use a few well-tried preparations, learning from experience what to expect of them. It is better to increase or reduce the dose of a single drug to obtain an appropriate response than to indulge in polypharmacy, changing repeatedly from one drug to another in the hope of better results.

The drugs listed below are suggested from experience such as this, but fashions change, and others may be preferred. However, this does not alter the principles that it is best to use as few drugs, and as little of them, as possible. Preference for tablets or elixirs varies.

Insomnia
Avoid barbituates. They have their uses in agitation and control of pain (q.v.) but have no place as hypnotics in old people owing to the risk of cumulative effects causing, instead of allaying, confusion and restlessness.

The following drugs may be tried: chloral hydrate 250–500 mg or dichlorphenazone (Chloralol) 325–650 mg.

Agitation
This varies from the late-afternoon restlessness, discontent, and wandering of some early dementias, to the nocturnal excursions of anxious patients searching for an outlet or object they cannot explain, or to more aggressive and violent reactions by day or by night. The difficulty is to

prescribe really effective medication from a long list of highly recommended drugs.

Avoid monoamine oxidase inhibitors. They have too many undesirable side-effects.

Use familiar phenothiazine derivatives.

There are three groups of chemically related compounds derived from the phenothiazine nucleus, all with differences in potency, clinical effects, side-effects and toxicities. For old people the most satisfactory preparations are the following.

Chlorpromazine (Largactil). Chlorpromazine has a central sedative action, and relieves agitation, restlessness, and disturbed behaviour. It is an antiemetic and, as it will potentiate the effects of hypnotics or analgesics, it may be combined successfully with them to keep down the dose and the risk of addiction and to control persistent vomiting in terminal illness. Its side-effects include tachycardia, diarrhoea, and skin photosensitivity. Amongst more serious *reactions* are:

1 allergic skin and mucosal conditions, especially of mouth (angular stomatitis and glossitis), pharynx, and larynx
2 hypotension: a sudden persistent drop in pressure, most liable to occur with intramuscular injections (which are also most painful)
3 hypothermia, which may occur even in moderately warm surroundings
4 dyskinesias, owing to blockade of dopaminergic transmission to the striatal receptors during prolonged chlorpromazine therapy or even after its use has been discontinued
5 toxic idiosyncrasies, including jaundice and blood dyscrasias

Beginning with 10 or 25 mg twice or three times a day the dose may be increased, but need rarely exceed a total of 150 mg daily because if this does not control behaviour disorder it is probably best to reduce the dose of chlorpromazine and add another sedative, e.g.:

chlorpromazine 25 mg	8 a.m.	2 p.m.	8 p.m.
chloral hydrate 250 mg	10 a.m.	4 p.m.	10 p.m.

Perphenazine (Fentazine: Trilafon). Mentioned only because it is safer and less painful by injection than chlorpromazine and is effective in quieting the noisy violence sometimes encountered in delirium or dementia with less risk of hypotension. Its most serious side-effect is parkinsonism, so that its use is probably best reserved for the few occasions when injections may be necessary. The dose in 2·5–5 mg intramuscularly.

Thioridazine (Melleril). This is sometimes more successful in controlling the agitated unhappiness of some elderly invalids than chlorpromazine.

Dosage varies from 25 to 75 mg two, three, or four times daily. Adverse reactions are similar to those of chlorpromazine.

Control of pain

Pain is subjective, endurance is variable, and fear in anticipation may be worse than the event. Individual response to analgesics is unpredictable, and dosage has to be flexible, titrated to individual need. Success in management is almost entirely a question of gaining and holding the patient's confidence: it may be lost for days owing to a single lapse into severe pain because of a missed or an ineffective dose. Even worse is the loss of dignity which is the right of a dying patient.

There are certain cardinal *rules of treatment*:

1 The patient's symptoms should be assessed with care, not only to make a diagnosis, but also to ascertain what the patient means by pain, and to make sure that other complaints adding to the misery are not overlooked. Mental distress is often worse than physical pain.
2 The character of the pain, its severity, how it is provoked, and its timing have to be determined.
3 Constant pain needs constant control:
    a appropriate analgesics should be given to prevent pain, not to suppress it after it strikes
    b if selection, dosage, and timing are right the patient should know *no* pain and yet retain awareness, consciousness, and peace of mind
    c the aim should be to ensure that the patient never has to ask for analgesia or be denied it when pain is irregular (i.e. because it is thought necessary to wait 'until the proper time')
    d the strongest opponent of effective analgesia is pain itself, aggravated by fear and tension
    e *per contra*, if it is shown that severe pain can be controlled, smaller doses become increasingly effective
    f pain associated with vomiting or with dyspnoea gives rise to some of the most difficult problems, and special efforts must be made to relieve these complications.

Addiction, called 'demanding dependence' by Saunders is a source of undignified unhappiness which is unnecessary in her long experience when the patient and the drugs are handled properly.

There are three categories of pain to consider.

Aches. Muscular and arthritic aches and other causes of discomfort which, although of no great pathological significance, may detract greatly from the patient's sense of well-being and respond only to an appropriate analgesic. Begin with caffeine–codeine compounds and progress to propoxyphene or to analgesics prescribed more specifically for arthritic pain such as phenylbutazone or naproxen. Distress which seems to be disproportionate to the source of pain may respond better to small supplements of phenothiazine derivatives than to increasing doses of analgesics: try chlorpromazine 10–25 mg, or methotrimeprazine (Nozinan) 10–50 mg. It may be necessary to resort to codeine (by mouth or by injection) or to morphine (see below).

Special pain. Special varieties of pain, important to pin-point, because they may respond so dramatically to specific treatment are:

1 *Polymyalgia rheumatica:* this a variant of giant-cell arteritis (p. 44) allied to temporal arteritis, characterized by prostration with disabling muscular pain in shoulder and pelvic girdles, outstanding dejection, the wretchedness of constitutional upset, and usually (but not always) an exceedingly high erythrocyte sedimentation rate of 100 or more. It responds dramatically to prednisone 30–50 mg daily as an initial dose, tapering at weekly intervals to a maintenance level of 7·5 mg daily by the fourth week which may have to be continued for some months.

2 *Post-hemiplegic epileptic pain:* spontaneous thalamic pain after strokes sometimes responds to small doses of phenobarbitone (30 mg twice daily) when analgesics are ineffective. It is thought that an epileptic focus may be the origin of the sensory disturbance in these patients.

3 *Trigeminal and post-herpetic neuralgias:* the severe pain sometimes associated with these conditions may respond to either carbamazepine (Tegretol) or to diphenylhydantoin (Dilantin). These drugs are anticonvulsants, but their effect in neuralgia is not necessarily central, be cause they also block peripheral transmission.

Intractable neurogenic, colicky, or metastatic bone pain. This category demands relief by opium derivatives because no non-habit-forming drugs are adequate. It may be possible to defer introducing them for continuous medication until the late stages of a fatal illness by good early management. Their use may then be restricted to a relatively brief period when a fatal outcome is clearly inevitable, and when their effectiveness outweighs the risks of addiction; or of respiratory depression and a diminished cough reflex. The most popular drug still is morphine hydrochloride 5–10 mg by hypodermic injection or in the Brompton cocktail: Rx morphine hydrochloride 15 mg, codeine phosphate 10 mg, gin (or rectified spirit) 10 ml, honey 5 ml, chloroform water 15 ml. Dose: 15–30 ml according to circumstances.

Levorphanol tartrate (Dromoran) 2–4 mg by injection or by mouth has similar properties to morphine but is more effective in small doses with more prolonged action.

Percodan (oxycodone–aspirin–caffeine compound) is intermediate in action between milder analgesics and opiates.

Meperidine HCl (Pethidine) 50–150 mg is given by mouth or by injection. Much less effective orally, it is an indifferent pain-reliever *except* in colic—especially renal colic, an agonizing pain which it relieves within minutes owing to its spasmolytic action.

Alcohol or prednisone 5–10 mg by mouth should be added if pain is complicated by depression unrelieved by imipramine.

Cyclizine (marzine) 50 mg by mouth is added if pain is complicated by vomiting.

Do everything possible to relieve the mental pain of unbearable dyspnoea.

'The art of giving analgesics is to keep them continually at the patient's own optimum dose.' With frail old people this usually means the use of paediatric doses. Know the drug, its effects, and side-effects; fit the dose to the patient; use it regularly to keep the pain in constant remission; and combine it when necessary with adjuvants that you know equally well.

It is a common, and unforgivable, error to withhold analgesics in the terminal patient. The merits of effective pain relief are inestimable; the risks of addiction minimal.

4 The use of drugs in geriatric medicine

There are two kinds of hazards in prescribing for old people: those which relate to methods of prescribing, and those caused by the susceptibility of old people to side-effects from drugs.

Prescribing methods

The steady output of new preparations, the persuasive advertising of drug firms, and the growing demands on medical services from an ageing population, combine to put heavy pressure on doctors to give medicines to old people which they may not need, or which may continue to be taken long after the need for them has passed. The *risks* which have been highlighted in various investigations of the use and abuse of drugs in geriatric medical practice include:

1 confusion and erratic use of medicines when an old person has too many to deal with efficiently
2 failing memory leading to missed doses or, perhaps worse, to the same dose being repeated
3 too much, or too little, medication because instructions are not clear and explicit
4 the tendency of old people to hoard surplus pills, to misuse outdated medicines, to try them out on other people, or to experiment with drugs borrowed from their friends
5 inadequate records causing duplication of prescriptions owing to consultation with different doctors, each unaware of the medicines prescribed by the others.

It may not be possible to impose patterns of prescribing which will eliminate hazards inherent, partly, in the make-up of old-agers, but it is possible to reduce them:

1 by meticulous routine check of drugs prescribed for old people
2 by avoiding prescription of any drugs for an old person until it is known what they happen to have already

3 by prescribing prepackaged drugs, each dose being marked with the day and the time it is to be taken
4 by observing two wise rules of geriatric medication recommended by Wade (1972):
  a never administer a drug without good reason
  b give as few drugs as possible at any one time

Adverse drug reactions

Reactions to drugs caused by individual idiosyncrasy (such as rashes or gastrointestinal upsets) or by drug interactions occur in old age as in earlier life, but there is an added risk in the elderly patient of susceptibility to reactions created by diminished reserves, which affect the distribution, the metabolism, and the excretion of drugs. Disorders of these may lead to the accumulation of higher plasma levels of drugs than would normally occur with the adult therapeutic dose, or to more prolonged drug action than in younger patients. Hurwitz (1969) showed that the incidence of adverse reactions to drugs is significantly higher in patients over 60 years of age and in women than in men. The profile of a patient at risk of adverse reactions outlined by Davison (1973) is a small elderly female, with a history of hay-fever, urticaria, or other allergic illness, with previous idiosyncrasy to some drug, with multiple complaints, and with renal or mental impairment.

Old people may be eccentric in their attitudes to taking the medicines they are given, but once taken, their absorption by mouth or through the intestinal tract is much the same as in younger adults. However, the *distribution* of drugs as they are absorbed may be influenced by circulatory insufficiency which alters the rate of recirculation through the liver and other tissues concerned in drug metabolism. Obesity or cachectic states affect distribution in that fat is a storage depot for lipid-soluble drugs; drug tolerance correlates to some extent with lean body mass.

Drugs are disposed of mainly in the liver by microsomal enzymatic oxidation, reduction, hydrolysis, or conjugation. There are no precise tests to estimate how much ageing affects hepatic capacity to metabolize, detoxicate, or dispose of the drugs recirculated through it, but these functions are as likely as those of any other system to be impaired by reduced efficiency and reserves.

Drugs eliminated by excretion are disposed of through the kidneys by glomerular filtration, by tubular secretion, or by tubular diffusion. Therefore, impaired renal function, a commonplace in old age, readily leads to intoxication, especially with drugs such as digitalis which are excreted unchanged by the kidneys.

Reduced intellectual capacity in some old people predisposes to disorientation and confusion in response to certain drugs, especially those used for sedation and relief of pain. Antihypertensive drugs (reserpine or methyldopa), digitalis, and barbituates often lead to depression and apathy. It is not always possible to anticipate these reactions, but they represent another aspect of poverty of reserves allied to hepatic and renal insufficiency, which necessitate caution in the drugs which are used for old people, and in the doses prescribed for them.

Some of the more commonly incriminated drugs, and the reactions to be expected, are these.

Antibiotics. Ampicillin was once notorious for morbilliform or erythematous rashes which accompanied or followed its use, more in old people than in children, for some unexplained reason. A modification in production has reduced this risk. Caution is necessary with streptomycin, kanamycin, and neomycin because of the risks of deafness or of renal failure. Chloramphenicol may cause marrow aplasia, and may upset the metabolism of some other drugs (e.g. tolbutamide). If used at all it should be used in moderation and be discontinued within a week.

Digitalis. Digitalis, especially when combined with a diuretic, is a 'potent source of adverse reactions' (Hurwitz), and heads the list of drugs causing them. Arrhythmias are common; nausea, vomiting, and slowing of the heart beat less so. Mental confusion, or an increased heart rate, also occur as side-effects but may not be recognized as symptoms of digitalis toxicity. The risk is increased by potassium deficiency and therefore by misuse of diuretics without potassium supplements. The adage 'once on digitalis, always on digitalis' is dangerous to apply in geriatric medical practice (Dall 1970; Davison 1973).

Atrial fibrillation in old age may be slow, intermittent, and symptomless until an episode of tachycardia or heart failure call for short-term treatment with small doses of digoxin and diuretics.

Anti-hypertensive therapy. There are probably more contraindications than indications for the treatment of patients over 70 years of age with antihypertensive drugs, especially guanethidine and other more potent agents. Hypotensive drugs may do more harm than good in old people who have symptoms of postural hypotension, who have had strokes, or have evidence of renal failure. If antihypertensive therapy is considered necessary in the treatment of left ventricular failure in an old ager, thiazide derivatives, with or without methyldopa, are the drugs to use.

Anticholinergic drugs and levadopa. The incidence of side-effects is high in the treatment of parkinsonism. Synthetic anticholinergic drugs cause visual disturbances or retention, and special care is necessary in patients with prostatic disease. Mental disturbances, hallucinations, and delirium also occur, and are a common indication of amantadine idiosyncrasy. Treatment with levadopa should be started cautiously with the smallest possible doses, given always with food. Multivitamin preparations which include pyridoxine must be avoided (pyridoxine reverses the antiparkinson effect of levadopa). The most common adverse effects are gastrointestinal, hypotensive, and mental (agitation, confusion, or psychotic behaviour) (see p. 63).

The side-effects of sedatives, tranquillizers, and analgesics have been mentioned in the section on terminal care, advising against the use of monoamine oxidase inhibitors.

Oral antidiabetic drugs. Adverse reactions to these are discussed on p. 69.

Drug interactions

The risk of these is increased in prescribing for old people because their multiple complaints often lead to multiple medicines. The list of possible actions of one drug upon another is immense (Melman and Morrelli 1972) varying from direct chemical or physical interactions to alterations in absorption, distribution, biotransformation, and excretion. Davison (1973) has described some of the more common interactions to be anticipated and avoided in geriatric clinical practice:

1 Tetracyline forms an inabsorbable complex with alkalies and with ferrous iron; the latter should be discontinued, therefore, if a patient requires oral tetracyclines.
2 Alkalies also reduce the absorption of weak acids such as salicylates and sulphonamide.
3 Drugs which are reversibly protein-bound may be displaced from binding sites by other competing drugs leading to alterations in therapeutic levels: e.g. phenylbutazone will displace sulphonamides (antidiabetic or antibacterial), and release action may cause hypoglycaemia in one instance, and enhance the effect or lead to toxic reactions in the other. Phenylbutazone, diphenylhydantoin, and salicylates are amongst the drugs that act similarly to displace warfarin and cause bleeding in patients on anticoagulant therapy.
4 Drugs that depend on binding to special receptor sites for their effect may prevent access of other agents to the receptors. Antihistamines, phenothiazines, and tricyclic antidepressants of the imipramine group, like atropine, block acetylcholine from its receptors and when combined may induce side-effects resembling atropine overdose. Phenothiazines and imipramine also block α-adrenergic receptors to cause hypotension.

5 Some drugs stimulate the metabolic enzyme systems and accelerate the breakdown of other drugs, e.g. chloral hydrate and meprobamate speed up the biotransformation of warfarin, phenytoin, phenylbutazone, and barbituates. If doses are increased to compensate, and the 'accelerator' is discontinued, overdosage may occur.

6 Other reactions inhibit drug metabolism. Tolbutamide hypoglycaemia and diphenylhydantoin toxicity have been attributed to inhibition of their metabolism by dicumarol, phenylbutazone, and salicylates.

7 Interactions from effects of previously administered drugs include digitalis toxicity attributable to potassium loss from previous thiazide therapy; the effect of thyroid therapy which necessitates increased barbiturate and digitalis dosage and decreased anticoagulants; and the effect of antibiotics on bowel flora which synthesize vitamin K and reduce warfarin requirements.

Despite the physician's best efforts to maintain detailed records, to check all drugs taken by his patients, and to keep up-to-date with clinical pharmacology, perhaps access to a computer program of known and of likely interactions, as suggested by Melman and Morrelli, will prove to be the most effective means of minimizing their dangers.

General points to remember

The following comments on 'Drugs in the elderly' come from Dr. J. P. Gemmell:

1 Plasma volume and extracellular fluids are decreased in old age, so drugs may reach high concentrations.

2 The liver excretes or metabolizes most drugs, and this function is impaired by ageing.

3 The ability of the kidney to excrete drugs decreases with age.

For these reasons average 'adult' doses may be excessively high, leading to cumulative effects.

'Polypharmacy is the curse of the elderly. Have them bring in *all* drugs they are taking or, better still, check their drug cupboards.'

5 Skin diseases common in old age

Susan M. Burge

Changes in ageing skin are listed in Table 1 (p. 10). There is individual variation in the appearance of the skin, and environmental factors such as sunlight, cold, and trauma are as important in aetiology as those that are inherited. Prolonged exposure to solar ultraviolet radiation causes wrinkling, drying, yellowing, inequalities of pigmentation, disordered keratinization, and loss of collagen with thickening and degeneration of remaining fibres. The role of sunlight in the origin of skin cancer is well-established. Deprivation may cause malnutrition or be associated with exposure and poor hygiene. Persistent cold exposure alters peripheral circulation with reactions such as ulcerated chilblains, acrocyanosis, and Raynaud's disease.

Intrinsic aetiological factors discussed by Verbov (1974) include peripheral vascular changes which alter responses to injury, infection, or cold; impaired sensory perception which blunts recognition of itching or pain; and impaired T- and B-cell functions causing a decline in the immune response. Genetic and endocrine factors may induce premature ageing of skin, and emotional upsets or psychiatric illness may initiate or prolong skin disease.

Presentation of skin disease in old age is often atypical and may be complicated by underlying systemic disorders, drug therapy, or social problems. Benign changes common in ageing skin are: *skin tags*, *seborrhoeic warts* (superficial brown, greasy, papules), *senile lentigines* (pigmented macules on exposed areas, especially on the backs of the hands), *sebaceous hyperplasia* (soft yellow papules on the forehead), *senile comedomes*, and *senile purpura* (on extensor surfaces of hands and arms or face and neck, from small skin vessels torn easily by minor trauma when their collagen and elastic fibre support is eroded by senile atrophy).

Tumours

The incidence of skin tumours is increased in the aged; clinical features vary, and biopsy is essential for diagnosis.

Keratoacanthoma. Keratoacanthoma is a benign tumour easily mistaken clinically and histologically for a carcinoma. It occurs on exposed skin as a nodular lesion with a central keratin plug. It grows far more quickly than a squamous cell carcinoma, reaching maximum size in about 6 weeks, and then resolves spontaneously leaving a deep scar. Early removal gives a better cosmetic result and the tissue can be sent for histological examination.

Solar keratoses. These are benign keratotic lesions on exposed skin which may progress to frank squamous cell carcinomata. They respond to early treatment with cryotherapy or topical 5-fluorouracil.

Intra-epidermal carcinoma.

1 *Bowen's disease:* presents usually on unexposed skin as a slow-growing, scaly, erythematous macule, which may have been mistaken for an eczematous or psoriatic lesion. The prognosis is good because Bowen's disease remains intraepidermal for a long time before becoming invasive. It responds well to cryotherapy, excision, or radiotherapy.
2 *Paget's disease of the nipple:* is easily mistaken for eczema. Therefore unilateral eczematous lesions of the nipple are always suspect and need biopsy. Intraepidermal carcinoma in this site is always associated with underlying adenocarcinoma and the treatment is mastectomy.

Basal cell carcinoma (rodent ulcer). This slow-growing, locally invasive tumour rarely develops metastases. It commonly presents on the face, at first as a small smooth nodule with a pearly, rolled edge, developing a superficial crusted ulcer in the centre as it grows. Superficial spreading basal cell carcinomata sometimes occur on the trunk producing erythematous plaques with a distinctive edge. The prognosis is excellent and lesions may be treated by radiotherapy, or by surgery.

Squamous cell carcinoma. This may occur on any site, including mucous membranes. There may have been a pre-existing lesion such as solar keratosis, varicose ulcer, or radiotherapy burn. Prognosis depends on the degree of differentiation. The poorly differentiated highly invasive tumour may have extended to regional lymph nodes before the patient presents. Excision or radiotherapy are the usual methods of treatment.

Hutchinson's lentigo. Hutchinson's lentigo is a large brown macule occurring on the face. It is benign but may undergo malignant melanomatous change. Lesions should therefore be watched for evidence of nodule formation, ulceration, or alteration in pigmentation. At this stage treatment is surgical and prognosis is better than other types of malignant melanoma.

Malignant melanoma. This is an uncommon skin tumour, fortunately, because prognosis is poor. It may arise from normal skin or from a pre-existing naevus. Subungual malignant melanoma may be mistaken for a haematoma.

Secondary carcinoma. Secondary carcinoma occurs only occasionally in the skin, most often from a primary in breast, lung, or kidney.

Pruritus

This is a common problem in old people whose skin is atrophic and dry. It may be exacerbated by obsessive cleanliness. It is important to exclude exogenous causes of itching:

1 Infestation with lice or fleas, especially in the recluse, and in other socially isolated and neglected old people.
2 Scabies may present atypically in elderly patients, with relatively little itching and very lichenified eczematous skin. The diagnosis is made by demonstrating the acarus.
3 Drug sensitivity.
4 Systemic disease: obstructive biliary disease, chronic renal failure, diabetes, hyperthyroidism, iron deficiency anaemia, polycythaemia, or malignancy, especially the reticuloses.

When itching is intense it may be necessary to start treatment before the diagnosis is confirmed. Oral antihistamines and a soothing topical preparation such as calamine lotion with 0·25–1% menthol may help. Nails may have to be cut and protective gloves or bandages provided, especially for confused elderly patients. Zinc paste with 1–2% phenol is an effective antipruritic for pruritis ani.

Eczema

Asteatotic eczema. The skin (especially on extensor surfaces) becomes dry and chapped, and eventually the stratum corneum fissures (*eczema craquele*). Elderly patients are particularly vulnerable and the condition is exacerbated by washing and by cold weather with a low humidity. Occasionally hypothyroidism or lymphoma may be aetiological factors. Simple treatment by reducing bathing and providing emollients is all that is necessary, e.g. ung. emulsificans as a soap substitute, oilatum emollient, aqueous cream.

Nummular (discoid) eczema. Erythematous and vesicular coin-shaped lesions occur, most frequently on the legs, often in association with dry skin. Treatment with emollients and tar preparations (3% liquor picis carbonis in aqueous cream) is useful, but the condition tends to be chronic and emotional tension may be an important factor causing it to persist.

Gravitational eczema. This eczema occurs over the lower legs and is usually secondary to chronic venous insufficiency. The skin may become lichenified, and there may be associated oedema, purpura, pigmentation, or ulceration. The principle of treatment is to restore the venous drainage of the leg. In mild cases elastic bandages may be sufficient. They should be applied from the toes to the knee before the patient gets up in the morning, and walking should be encouraged. If itching is troublesome occlusive coal-tar bandages beneath a support bandage may help, renewed at intervals of 10 days. Topical steroids may be needed in the acute stages. Obese patients should be encouraged to lose weight. Contact dermatitis caused by medicament sensitization is a common complication.

Seborrhoeic eczema (dermatitis). The cause of this common condition is not known but prevalence is increased in the elderly. The eruption occurs on the scalp and forehead, symmetrically behind the ears, and in the auditory meatus, in the eyebrows, on the cheeks, and in naso-labial folds. There is dull erythema with a greasy scale. The rash may also involve presternal and interscapular regions, the umbilicus, and flexures. Blepharitis is a frequent association. Secondary infection with candida or pathogenic bacteria is common. Topical steroid antiseptic ointments (Vioform-HC), sulphur-containing creams (2% Salicylic acid + 2% sulphur in. aqueous cream), and tar shampoos are useful.

Intertrigo. Intertrigo occurs in flexural regions where skin surfaces rub together. It is a common problem in obese, unhygienic, immobile, or incontinent patients. Important contributing factors are perspiration, maceration by urine or faeces, and secondary infection (candida or bacteria). It must be differentiated from tinea, seborrhoeic dermatitis, and psoriasis. Infection should be treated and diabetes excluded. Skin surfaces should be separated and wet antiseptic dressings applied. Absorbent dusting powders (Zeasorb) and antiseptic drying agents such as gentian violet may be helpful.

Tinea pedis

Fungal infection of the foot (athlete's foot) is common. The infection usually starts in the toe clefts, causing scaling, maceration, and fissuring. It may spread to the soles where it can be confused with psoriasis or eczema. In any doubtful case scrapings should be taken for microscopy and culture. Occasionally maceration is caused by excessive perspiration alone. Mild cases, localized to the fourth toespace may respond to a simple absorbent powder (Zeasorb). Topical antifungal agents (miconazole) are effective, but recurrences are common. Extensive infection may require treatment with oral griseofulvin (500 mg per day for 4–6 weeks).

Herpes zoster

Occurs most often in patients over 50 years of age. There may be paraesthesiae and pain for some days before the appearance of a uni-lateral vesicular rash on an erythematous background, in the distribu-tion of a dermatome. The virus is thought to remain latent in the dorsal root ganglion to be re-activated in conditions associated with depressed immunity: in old age, by radiotherapy, by cytotoxic drugs, or by malignancy. Treatment with 20% idoxuridine in dimethyl sulphoxide on gauze, applied to fresh lesions for 3–4 days, decreases the incidence of post-herpetic neuralgia.

Rosacea

This is a chronic disorder of unknown aetiology which appears on the face in middle age. Erythema and telangiectasia affect nose, cheeks, and forehead in discrete or more confluent patches with or without an acneform eruption of papules, pustules, and nodules. Overgrowth of nasal soft tissue sometimes causes rhinophyma. It is associated with blepharitis, conjunctivitis, episcleritis, and keratitis. There is no specific treatment for the erythema other than avoidance of causes of vaso-dilation (heat, hot food, and liquids, alcohol), but 2% sulphur in aqueous cream is palliative, and the acneform eruption responds to low doses of a broad-spectrum antibiotic (tetracycline 250 mg b.d.). Topical corticosteroids make rosacea worse.

Leg ulcers

These may be venous (gravitational), arterial (ischaemic), mixed vascular, or of neuropathic origin.

Gravitational leg ulcers. Gravitational ulcers are associated with deep venous incompetence often attributable to previous thrombosis. The victims are often immobile and obese. Venous drainage is impaired and prolonged stasis results in pigmentation, eczema, and obliteration of cutaneous vessels, producing small atrophic white scars (*atrophie blanche*). The skin is very vulnerable and minor trauma causes ulcers, usually on the lower third of the legs above the medial malleolus.

Patients may have tried various topical preparations and the incidence of medicament allergy amongst them is high. Contact dermatitis as a complication may delay healing and a patch test is indicated if this is suspected. Healing may also be delayed by anaemia or vitamin deficiency.

Large, oozing ulcers should be treated, initially, with the leg elevated, applying wet dressings of half-strength eusol changed two or three times daily. The old-fashioned system of eusol irrigations within a loose-fitting polythene 'stocking' works admirably, and avoids the discomfort of having to remove dried dressings from an extensive raw area. Anaemia and other contributory deficiencies should be corrected. An oral antibiotic may be required when an ulcer is complicated by cellulitis. Topical antibiotics should not be used owing to the risk of contact dermatitis.

When the ulcer is clean an occlusive dressing changed once a week will encourage both healing and mobility. An elastic or crepe bandage overlying a Viscopaste or Quinaband support bandage should be applied carefully to give support, but not painful constraint, to the leg. Treatment may be necessary for months to heal a large ulcer, and pinch grafts may have to be used occasionally. Once healed, continued support from elastic stockings and constant vigilance to avoid injury are essential. Topical steroids are contraindicated unless there is contact dermatitis. They delay healing and prolonged use causes skin atrophy adding to the risk of further ulceration.

Arterial ulcers. Ulcers arising from arterial insufficiency are painful, punched out, and associated with other symptoms and signs of ischaemia (claudication, absent peripheral pulses, and shiny cool skin). Elevation, occlusive bandages, and vasodilators are contraindicated because they may further compromise the circulation.

Neuropathic ulcers may be associated with diabetes, alcoholism, tabes dorsalis, or leprosy. They tend to be deeply penetrating and there is frequently underlying osteomyelitis, so radiology is always indicated.

Blistering disorders

Blisters are often traumatic, from hot-water bottles, friction burns, or pressure. Other causes include drugs (barbiturates), prolonged stasis with much oedema, contact dermatitis, infection (herpes simplex or zoster), and pemphigoid.

Bullous pemphigoid. This is seen mainly in the over-sixties. The patient develops tense, symmetrical, sub-epidermal bullae which are often haemorrhagic. They occur mainly on the limbs and lower abdomen. There may be erythematous macules and occasional oral ulceration. The blisters rupture and the skin heals rapidly. Detection of auto-antibodies to basement membrane confirms the diagnosis. The disease is relatively benign and responds rapidly to oral prednisolone (60 mg/day). Azathioprine is used to reduce the amount of steroid necessary. Steroids are tailed off once blisters have stopped appearing, but maintenance therapy may be required for several years.

6 Home assessment visits

E. W. Knox

Introduction

Each home assessment visit in geriatric medical practice is a unique challenge, most satisfying to an interested physician and, when properly accomplished, an excellent therapeutic procedure. The physician, having escaped from his white coat, wards, and out-patient clinic, is able to 'play away', whereas patients and their relatives on their 'home ground' display more confidence and are more forthright in presenting their problems.

A social worker is a valuable adviser to a physician on a visit, and her contribution cannot be replaced by bringing the patient to a clinic with a social work report, but the physician shares responsibility with the social worker in recognizing significant environmental factors relating to the presenting medical problems—for example, objects kept on a high shelf as the possible source of falls in a patient thought to have vertebral basilar insufficiency, or collapsed springs and a sagging mattress preventing a parkinsonian patient from turning in bed.

Environment

Standing in the rain studying the faded paint flaking from a front door and listening to an elderly invalid shuffle slowly and painfully along the hall in response to a knock makes one more aware of the domestic difficulties that beset our patients. The ominous sound of a fall behind the closed door is an unhappy introduction to a visit, and one must have the patience to wait and allow time for an over-anxious or flustered person to answer. For a patient who is liable to fall a quiet, tree-lined avenue, with few pedestrians and cars, does not offer the voluntary supervision evident in a street where the arrival of the visiting doctor prompts neighbours to emerge, ostensibly to examine the sky or to clean a window. A house in a busy street may be conveniently close to shops and the Post Office, but risks are self-evident if the patient is dementing and wanders. If the door has been left open, or a key is available on a string reached through the letter box, it is reassuring to let the patient know 'this is the doctor coming' as one goes along the hall or up the stairs. One hesitates to call if window blinds are drawn; it is better to inquire next door and to learn that the patient to be visited has died than to risk embarrassment for everyone—including the family doctor who may have been unable to cancel the visit in time.

Furniture

In a household with restricted floor space a patient whose balance is precarious has little scope for walking practice, but finds reassurance in moving around by holding on to familiar items of furniture. (This is referred to as going 'by the grips', 'by the catches', or 'by the hoults'.) A Zimmer walking aid on top of a wardrobe, in a back yard, or pushed between the rails of the stairs may pay tribute to the willingness of nurses, social workers, or doctors to help, but suggests a lack of accurate home assessment. Falls at home may be 'cushioned' by an armchair or settee or a wall, in contrast to hospital experience where a patient may crash full-length on a vast expanse of floor and possibly fracture femur or pelvis.

A patient who has difficulty in rising from a chair may obtain one tailor-made to a suitable leg length, or an ejector seat, but before this is used a short session of training is essential. Patients who have no insight into their frailty and 'take off' unsupervised are a constant source of anxiety and may be safer in a low chair, perhaps substituting a thinner cushion for the seat of a settee or comfortable armchair. The Offerton chair with a table-front is widely used, but we are all familiar with the geriatric Houdini, a potential limbo-dancing prize-winner, for whom the best solution is freedom to walk around with as much supervision as can reasonably be supplied behind a locked door. Most elderly people prefer to live dangerously in their own homes rather than exist safely—but unhappily—under institutional care.

A patient who requires a high chair with an arm-rest will also require a raised toilet-seat and hand-grips. The same criteria apply to the indispensable bedside commode, best placed in a corner of the bedroom between the bed and the wall to give support so that the patient can only fall forwards. The Renway bed commode has variable-height legs and bed attachments which make transfer from bed to commode relatively easy and safe.

Bed height is important, both to the patient, if it is too high to get in and out safely; and to the relatives or district nurse if it is too low. An inch or two sawn off wooden legs, or blocks below them, may make all the difference to the patient's independence or to back-breaking nursing care.

An extra hand-rail and improved lighting are often needed on stairs, but patients who cannot negotiate them may have to be persuaded to accept a move to a ground-floor room (usually with a commode) to avoid becoming completely housebound. Failure to have made the change earlier, or to obtain it at all, need not surprise the visiting physician—the reluctant recluse may not realize that bathroom facilities can be improvized downstairs, or may wish to avoid intrusion into the ground-floor social life of a crowded household, transforming a precariously controlled situation into a family crisis.

Fires

Old people do not take kindly to fire guards. Unfortunately a fine-mesh, spark-proof guard traps heat and may only be on show at appropriate times to please a home-help, district, nurse or other visitor. A large-mesh guard may prevent a patient falling into the fire, but it is cumbersome and not sparkproof. The tea caddy and other necessities should not be kept on the mantelpiece. A dull, slow-moving patient in a cold room 'heated' by a glimmer of a fire, signals the need for immediate action to forestall the onset of coma, cold axillae, and the 'lump of lard' appearance of hypothermia.

Relatives

A home visit is an opportunity to meet and assess others besides the patient: relatives, if there are any, neighbours, or other visitors responsible for the old person in one way or another. A private talk with them can be most helpful, covering what they know of the patient's illness and disability, details of the 24-hour routine (sleep, toilet needs at night, washing, nursing, and the range of activity, aided or unaided). They may be surprised to be asked about the patient's preferences in reading, radio or TV programmes, but it is important to know about these if special arrangements have to be made to satisfy the patient's needs at home or, even more so, in hospital. Details of eating habits, medication, and idiosyncrasies are important too if a patient with a 'poor swallow', used to purées, is to avoid being choked by solid food in hospital; or if faecal impaction is to be prevented by an accustomed laxative. Inquiry about idiosyncrasies may prompt a relative to recall drug sensitivity which the patient has long forgotten.

Arrangements for cooking, laundry, household chores, shopping, and dependence on help from relatives or others can be elicited by the social worker while the physician examines the patient.

This preliminary discussion, however brief, usually reveals the attitude of the relatives to the problems the patient presents. It varies from those who intend to continue looking after the patient and only seek assurance that all that can be done is being done, to others who seem to expect the visiting physician to remove the patient (and their problems) there and then in his car. Between these extremes are the willing majority who need advice, help from social services or supporting hospital facilities (out-patient investigation or day hospital care), or admission of the patient for assessment, rehabilitation, or continuing care. An example is the respite needed for a daughter who has given up her work and holidays for twelve years to look after her mother. If not suggested already by a social worker, nurse, or family doctor, the idea of temporary admission of the patient to give her daughter a holiday might be mentioned. However, anyone who has given up so much on behalf of a frail invalid must understand the risks of moving her to hospital—confusion from the change to strange surroundings, and cross-infection. It is not unusual for confusion leading to dehydration and more confusion to be followed by sedation, immobility, and a fatal broncho-pneumonia. An explanation of these risks may prevent the daughter from blaming herself for having 'killed my mother for a holiday'. If intermittent admissions are planned relatives must understand that relief for others depends on their integrity in meeting the discharge date agreed when the patient is admitted. Short-term admissions for investigation or rehabilitation do not present problems, but if there is to be delay in admission for continuing care this must be explained.

Drugs

Unnecessary medication, improper dosage, drug interactions, and adverse reactions are so commonplace in geriatric medical practice that a detailed outline of current drug therapy is an essential part of an assessment visit.

Many elderly patients would do better if essential drugs were taken in the proper dose at the proper time. Polypharmacy is the besetting weakness of much geriatric medication, and sometimes old people produce a receptacle filled with bottles and pill boxes. If a patient lives alone and is responsible for his own treatment, he must be able to read the labels, to understand and remember instructions, and to have the physical ability to administer and swallow medicines from various containers. These should be inspected to make sure that tablets have not become mixed by being spilled and returned to the wrong box. For a patient with poor memory, tablet-taking should be linked to a recurrent daily event: 'Take a blue tablet with your porridge in the morning and with your Horlicks at night' is more likely to be remembered than 'take a blue tablet morning and evening'. In those who are physically or mentally incapable of responsible medication, supervision of drug administration and of actual swallowing must be accepted by a relative, neighbour, home-help, or area warden.

The patient

The techniques of listening and talking to patients have been described by Fletcher (1980) and his advice applies equally, or even more, to interviews with aged than with younger people. It helps to set a patient at ease if the doctor, having shaken hands when introduced, sits at the bedside or makes physical contact with a friendly hand on the shoulder. Conversation should be slow and distinct, but not too loud, except to overcome real deafness. The object is to confirm the patient's complaints, avoiding too many tiring questions. Patient and relative may see the same situation very differently; a wife may complain of being worn out helping her husband to the lavatory at nights, without mentioning his pain; or a man complain he is 'in agony', without reference to his wife's exhaustion. Pain may be overlooked by the attendants of a mentally impaired geriatric patient, who may still be able to acknowledge it in answer to a direct question.

Mental assessment

The insiduous onset of senile (Altzeimer's) dementia is so slow that relatives constantly attending the patient may fail to appreciate the change and are genuinely convinced that he is mentally clear. It may be embarrassing to ask the simple questions of a mental assessment (and to protect a patient from being prompted by the onlookers), but a methodical check should be made of orientation, comprehension, concentration, and recent memory. The answers will give corresponding evidence of attentiveness, mood, behaviour, insight, and initiative.

This estimate of mental capacity is just as important as the examination of physical, central nervous, cardiovascular, or respiratory functions. It may be the critical factor in deciding whether a patient is capable of effective response to rehabilitation, or is impaired by inability to grasp what is being asked of him or to remember and concentrate on appropriate action. It may indicate paranoid tendencies or depression; it may distinguish the affable, kindly personality, acceptable everywhere, from the aggressive intolerance of the social outcast; or it may elicit the first vagaries of the patient who will progress to confused wandering, who cannot be coped with at home, to whom a cot-side is a challenge and every door an invitation, and whose safety demands a secure building, and the freedom to wander that alone gives them happiness. Questionnaires can give quantitative values of brain performance for such patients, but do not show what functions are good or bad. Knowledge of this, of personality, and of eccentricity is essential to ensure appropriate care when hospital admission follows home assessment.

Physical assessment
Many old people when visited are sitting at their firesides fully dressed, and unless there is good reason to embark on what may be a complex undressing exercise, one may have to be content with an assessment from clinical observation, and from tests of posture, balance, and walking patterns.

One does not have to be an exceptionally good noticer (p. 25) to spot the short neck and kyphosis of osteoporosis or spinal arthritis; the unblinking impassive expression, flexed head, and torticollis of parkinsonism; the smooth brow of some hypothyroid patients; the slack skin and loose collar of malignancy; the various complexions—cream, strawberries-and-cream, daffodil tint, malar flush, and spider naevi; the suffused eyes of an alcoholic and of polycythaemia; conjunctival pallor; asymmetrical naso-labial folds and degrees of ptosis; scleral, pupillary, and iris abnormalities; the degree of skin ageing; senile purpura and malignant skin lesions; venous lakes on lips; the ulnar deviation of normal ageing and of rheumatoid disease; other arthritic deformities of hands and wrists; the parkinsonian hand; or the beta-blocker cold hand.

If a patient has recently stopped eating or refused medication, examination of teeth, gums, tongue, and pharynx may reveal loose or carious teeth, ulcers related to these, to ill-fitting dentures, or to oral Cetiprin (emepronium bromide), or perhaps a malignant lesion.

If physically able, the patient should be asked to stand up from chair or bed and to walk across the room, with help if necessary. It is best for the visiting physician himself to give this, standing behind the patient and giving support with a hand in each axilla, or in front with the patient's forearms resting on his own supinated hands and forearms so that each can grasp the other's elbows. This gives a more accurate estimate of the patient's balance and postural control than watching at a distance, and makes it easier to assess a disorder of gait (pp. 50–3). It is also a guide to advice on the kind of help the patient or relatives may need to anticipate mishaps owing to unsteadiness and liability to falls.

Instruction may be needed in the proper way to get out of a chair (pulling the feet in and bending the body forward over them), in the use of walking aids—to *lean* on them (a point seldom stressed), or in methods of walking practice for the unreliable 'backslider' (pp. 51 and 65).

The question to ask yourself before leaving the house is: 'Why was I asked to see this patient?' Sometimes the relatives were dissatisfied with the patient's progress (or lack of it) and the family doctor has simply invited another opinion to reinforce his own assessment that no more can be done and the patient is best where he is. More often the visit originated in change—either in the patient's condition or in the support available to him. Occasionally it will be because someone from outside (perhaps a close relative on a trans-Atlantic sentimental journey) takes an objective view of what is thought to be a stable and satisfactory routine, and demands investigation.

The options available to the physician are:

1 to give the reassurance and support required by the family doctor. The physician, or the social worker, may suggest appliances, facilities, or the support of domiciliary services that appear to have been over-looked

2 out-patient investigation followed by home treatment

3 urgent admission for a medical or surgical emergency

4 admission as soon as possible for rehabilitation owing to a permanent handicap such as parkinsonism, a stroke, or arthritis

5 relief admission, usually arranged as a respite for the relatives of completely dependent patients, often as a prelude to cyclical 'intermittent' admissions of 4–6 weeks in and 4–6 weeks out, less commonly as a move towards continuing hospital care

6 to refer the patient to a more appropriate service: perhaps for the psychiatric care needed by a paranoid trouble-maker, or for the sheltered housing or residential care due to an infirm old ager in a hopelessly unsuitable household

The action to be taken may be agreed in discussion with the social worker as the visit ends. If the family doctor is present a decision may be made there and then, but if not the relatives must understand that he will be consulted immediately (in an emergency), or within the next 24 hours at most, and that he will decide with them what arrangements are to follow.

Finally, the findings on the visit are entered on a form of similar size to the hospital notes (Appendix 2) to be kept with the patient's hospital record.

7 Retirement

Regard old age as one of the bad habits
which a busy man has no time to form.
(Sir Adolph Abrahams)

The retired population of the United Kingdom is expected to exceed 10 million by 1981, and there has been a vast change in the proportion of elderly dependants to wage earners since the beginning of the century. In Great Britain in 1901, 61 per cent of men aged 65 and over were employed. By 1951 this figure was halved, at 31 per cent, and it is now only 18 per cent. The basis of these statistics may have varied at different censuses, and in the earlier years they were biased by a preponderance of workers in agriculture whose employment was long-continued, if not perpetual (Amulree 1951), but even if strict comparisons are compromised, the trend is obvious and we have almost reached a level of one retired person to every three in paid employment.

This immense increase in 'leisure years' is the result of improved life expectancy combined with the policies of compulsory and early retirement which have been adopted from the state services by the professions, commerce, and industry. It is a challenge to the national economy and society and the concern it has aroused is evident in the variety of statutory and voluntary institutions and programmes available to older workers preparing for or beginning their retirement. Details of these may be obtained from Pensions and National Insurance Offices or from Age Concern publications in the United Kingdom, and there are descriptions of research studies, medical social aspects, and resources in textbooks of geriatric medicine. There are also two splendid treatises on the philosophy of retirement, one written by an anonymous country doctor (1964); the other an anthology of essays on middle-age edited by Sir Heneage Ogilvie (1962).

Pre-retirement courses usually include hints on physical health which may apply generally to all those who are growing old, but one cannot generalize in the same way about mental outlook on retirement. Attitudes and reactions to it are wholly personal, peculiar to each individual, and influenced, amongst other factors, by the job he does and where he does it, by where and how he lives, and by his relationships with his family, friends, and fellow-workers. It would be interesting to know how retirement affects different groups of working people and to compare, for example, the reactions of men with those of women, the self-employed with the employees of big business or nationalized industry, the professions with commerce, or executives with the shop floor, but a basis for such comparisons would be difficult to devise, and reliable data would be even more difficult to obtain. Therefore, it is probably best not to presume to 'advise' too much in pre-retirement courses, but to set out thoughts to provoke discussion and constructive thinking amongst those who attend. What follows is a personal view of how the implications of present retirement policies and aspects of health in old age might be used in this way, a view which applies mainly to men and is based more on surmise than fact.

Attitudes to retirement

Excluding those who retire owing to ill-health, there are three groups of older workers approaching retirement: those who welcome it because they have cultivated so many outside interests and adjusted their way of life so successfully to make the most of them that it is a pleasure to retire; those who are able and anxious to continue at work; and those eager to retire because their job has become intolerable and they long to escape from it even more than they desire a rest or a change. The first group is self-sufficient but each of the others presents problems.

The incentives which encourage some people to continue working (or perhaps to resent being retired) vary. Some have no alternative interests; some enjoy the prestige of their seniority as much as the rewards and privileges that go with it; others 'with the work habit in their bones' feel deprived if they do not go on applying the skills and craftsmanship of many years of experience; and yet others will continue even if unfit, because they need the money. For such people compulsory retirement may bring serious losses—of status, income, companionship, independence, and of mental and physical activity. Some react badly, feeling deprived, losing self-respect, or considering themselves rejected by society. Others, however, who have stayed at work long after they were able for it may benefit by enforced retirement, and some studies have shown that, far from having an adverse effect on health, many people feel the better of it.

The third group, those who wish to retire more as an escape from undesirable work than to a more pleasurable life, suffer from what Sheppard (1981) describes as 'mid-career malaise'. This is a state of mind reached by increasing numbers of people whose quality of life at work has deteriorated, they have lost their job-satisfaction, or they have lived so long with a particular job that they have become 'demotivated from it'. Employers have gone some way towards recognizing this in occupations which are physically heavy, high risk, or intrinsically dissatisfying, by offering early retirement. (This may be enforced also to dispose of the 'burned out' manager, the 'obsolete' employee, or the person said to have 'plateaued in his mid-fifties'. Then it is either a misused administrative convenience, or an essential of efficient management, depending on the point of view.)

Older workers are said to be more content at work than young people, but this does not mean that those who stick to a particular occupation for many years necessarily become increasingly satisfied with it. On the contrary, they may be far from happy, but may have had no opportunity to make a change or to take time off to learn new skills—a primary cause of declining job satisfaction in Sheppard's experience. Even those who can pick and choose may be locked into their work by a superannuation scheme; the insurance company behind this becomes 'the arbiter of the worker's destiny' (Mackintosh 1954), encouraging the younger employee to hold on with the promise of retirement at a fixed age and with greater security, but operating against the interests of the restless middle-aged worker who cannot risk a move to a new job at an age when domestic expenses are high, and chances of entering another occupation for the first time are low.

Compulsory retirement at a fixed age must be both a convenience and a necessity in most occupations if only to ensure promotion where it is due, and to create a constant intake of youth, initiative, and new ideas. Ideally, middle-age (between 45 and 65 years old?) should be a time to change gear and to become engaged, at a slower pace is necessary, in new interests and activities at work. Compulsory retirement would be more acceptable if coupled in advance with an option into alternative work offering these attractions under less demanding conditions. Working continuity is important because, once retired, the will to begin a regular working routine again may soon be absorbed into other interests or blissful idleness. There is more wishful thinking than reality in the longing for re-employment sometimes expressed by pensioners. No large willing pool of potential workers is to be found amongst them. Undeniably the pool exists—it is the willingness that is in doubt (Amulree, 1951). For the same reason those who really want to find a use for their experience and skills after they retire do well to arrange a definite job beforehand. Otherwise their enthusiasm may wane while awaiting offers of employment that may never turn up.

For reasons discussed below, the older worker is wise to move from jobs where fast performance is essential, because he may still be able to learn and do well with tasks where care and accuracy are more important than speed. It should be possible to devise tests of capacity for manual workers wishing to make such a change, and to define for them criteria of pre-retirement or retirement jobs, giving the stronger man work within his stamina, and protecting the weaker from competition in an occupation beyond his physical powers. Welford (1954) thought the problem was to specify work for the elderly 'on which they can be employed whole-time, at economic rates, without special allowances, and with full use of their skilled capacity'. This is true for the manual worker, but pre-retirement plans must take account of another, greater, problem: the distinction between employees in physical labour and those in occupations which make their demands on the mind.

Mackintosh observed that the outstanding difference between the manual and the mental worker is the capacity for the latter to do harm, because while the product of most manual labour is good, the results of mental exertion can be disastrous. Yet, the mental worker approaching the threshold of retirement has often reached a level where his opportunities to do ill are extensive, and 'there is no one in a position to tell him to go home'. In the same vein Kennedy (1957) commented on the difficulties arising in the professions and management with the senior individual who is less concerned about salary than status, who has a vested interest in preventing change that might bring progress but would demand too much of his failing grasp of affairs, and who is reluctant to move if it means giving way to a more able junior and stepping down to a less prestigious post. Mackintosh said he always listened carefully to an elderly man who protested: 'I am as good as ever I was', for that was one of the earliest signs of declining mental powers: 'the dear man has begun to whistle in the growing intellectual dusk'. If anything were needed to justify compulsory retirement, lack of insight and complacent obtuseness of this kind would provide it.

These views were expressed in essays written long before the introduction into industry of the micro-chip, and it is difficult to predict whether this will make things easier or more difficult for the ageing employee. The impact of micro-electronics on all kinds of employment may have far-reaching effects on future policies for the older worker. A vast increase is anticipated in leisure time in a world where, apparently, people expect to be paid more and more money to give less and less time to work. There should be more opportunities in future for fulfilment and a worth-while contribution to society in creative craftsmanship of one kind or another, in the so-called 'care' services, and in a wide range of service industries; but to match progress and make the best use of available talent will call for a blueprint based on imaginative and painstaking planning, and for the education of co-operative participants. This could be encouraged by extending the scope of pre-retirement programmes such as those set up since 1959 by the Glasgow Retirement Council (Anderson 1980).

Faced with the prospect of retirement at a fixed age, many employees need encouragement to plan well ahead, to make the social contacts they will need in later years where they intend to settle, and to develop creative interests. Crafts and hobbies alone may not fill this need, and may not even appeal to people who would prefer to use their knowledge and experience in some intellectual activity. They may plan a new vocation in part-time employment or voluntary endeavour on behalf of the community, through church, social services, or Workers' Educational Association. There is scope for this even in the smallest village. The keynote should be to foster *involvement* (as distinct from employment) in local activities (G. M. Komrower 1980, personal communication), to avoid the risk that some run of becoming isolated in retirement, especially those who have moved to a new neighbourhood.

Employers and institutions may help, not only with the opportunities to change jobs mentioned earlier, but with training and facilities to take advantage of them, and by arranging free time or night classes for pre-retirement counselling. Special efforts may have to be made to attract the less out-going workers who may most need guidance. Voluntary pre-retirement classes seem to attract the more responsible, gregarious, intelligent, and enterprising employees, especially women—people who have less need of advice than of opportunities to use their talents. However, counselling is still worthwhile if it helps them to use these better in retirement on their own behalf or for others.

Perhaps these reflections apply only to those who by happy chance are born with the desire to develop aptitudes, acquire skills, extend their interests, and, throughout their lives, are constantly driven by a restless urge to engage in creative activity. There must be countless thousands of others with no such ambition who ask no more of life in retirement than food, fluids, warmth, and companionship—the cornerstones of survival mentioned at the beginning of this book. These must still be available to the fortunate people who live in small communities of towns and villages, but the all-important element of companionship is going, or has gone, from the cities where the friendly relationships of small street 'village life' have been broken up by inner city and high-rise development. Relatives and good neighbours are scattered, small shops, pubs, and clubs have been destroyed, and industrial conurbations must house many anxious, isolated pensioners who need friendship and help more than counselling.

Ageing and performance

Higher faculties and intellect hold up well against advancing age unless undermined by ill-health, but even those who escape pathological damage and are as fit and able as Sheldon's 'aristocracy of old age' must reconcile and adjust themselves to altered mental and physical performance in response to the structural and biochemical age changes described earlier (pp. 2, 23, 24 and Table 1). The effects of these changes on intellectual and physical activities have been studied by psychologists for many years, and the wellbeing of the older worker has attracted their special interest. This research and theories derived from it have been described by Bromley (1978) and Welford (1981) whose work should be consulted for detail. Only brief reference to some of their conclusions can be made here.

Bromley emphasizes the distinction to be made between *intellectual attainment* (maximum intellectual capacity) and *intellectual performance*. The first is an endowment realized by most people between the ages of 16 and 20; the second is a measure of ability to use intellect which depends on factors such as personal qualities and aptitudes, specialist knowledge and experience, technical skills, or even luck and good connections. Despite evidence of some decline with age, if intellect is constantly used to capacity it holds up well, especially vocabulary, information, and comprehension. Deterioration follows disuse, and may follow illness even more rapidly.

The outstanding mental change attributed to ageing is less efficient short-term memory. As people grow older they become slower to learn, slow to remember, and slower on the uptake with abstract ideas and reasoning. This is evident in tests which require them to assimilate and apply new information rather than old familiar knowledge. It explains the apparent rigidity of outlook and behaviour of old people who rely on standardized patterns of thought and action.

Data to be interpreted, learned, and remembered must first be perceived, then passed through the intracerebral processes necessary for identification, recognition, registration, reasoning, and initiation of appropriate reactions. It seems that what is perceived is first transmitted to a primary (short-term) memory store which can hold only three or four items at a time. As more information reaches the store these first items are lost unless they have been transferred to be retained in a secondary store equivalent to long-term memory. Failing memory in old age is attributed to failure to establish data in this secondary holding bank. The main problem is in initial perception and registration rather than in retention and retrieval. The explanation given for this is that either incoming sensory signals are weak, or that intracerebral processing is unsettled by 'neural noise'—spontaneous, random, neural activity which increases with age and has been shown to make fine discrimination less accurate in older people (Welford 1981).

These findings help to explain some limitations faced by those approaching retirement. In the arts, the law, finance, and similar activities it is possible to continue working successfully into old age, drawing upon knowledge and experience of concepts acquired in early professional education, but the scientist's intellectual productivity (in terms of original work) is usually maximal in his thirties, because it depends more on mastering and applying new concepts quickly and precisely to complex problems. Ageing manual workers may be slow to pick up a new skill, but given time, willingness, and work within their physical powers, they will succeed. Their performance may be slower than in youth, but it will probably be more consistent, more painstaking, and more accurate.

Physical condition is maintained at remarkably good levels by many old people who believe in moderate living and regular exercise. However, sooner or later most of them begin to feel the effects of cell loss which thins out some tissues (especially the irreplaceable cells of brain and muscle), and of loss of elasticity in others. Besides being unable to see or hear as well as in youth, their muscular strength is weakened, action is slower, and they are more easily tired. Almost all movement, from the most precise use of hand and arm to the reflex responses concerned with posture and balance, are reactions to sensory information transmitted to the brain from eye, ear, skin, muscles, and joints. Age brings failing eyesight, impaired hearing, and blunting of touch and position sense, and the ageing brain has to compensate for less accurate sensory input and for its reduced capacity to identify the incoming information, analyse it, match it against stored memories, and apply the conclusions drawn from this in appropriate action. Muscle activity is slower and weaker (reduced 25 per cent by age 60); joints are stiffened, with limitation of movement; postural control and balance are impaired; and confidence in precision movements is lessened because timing and performance have become irregular and jerky instead of co-ordinated and smooth.

Evidence of this decline appears in the fifties, the time to begin making adjustments and to anticipate stepping down to lower levels of activity. Most people retain the intellectual capacity to compensate for their deficiencies for many years if they have the good fortune also to retain the insight to use it. Pre-retirement courses can help, encouraging them to look at these problems in relation to their own circumstances, to adopt a way of life less restricted by former commitments, to become less consciously competitive than former social or working status may have demanded, and to develop the reliable habits and discretion they may need increasingly as time passes.

Health in retirement

Pre-retirement courses usually include a talk on health to explain age changes in mental and physical activities and how best to adjust to them.

Health in old age means more than freedom from disease. Few old people escape disorders of some kind or other, but fortunately most of them keep fit, active, and cheerful within the limits imposed by their disabilities and retain their independence as best they can. 'Health' in this sense includes a feeling of wellbeing and takes account of capability, and it depends on personal make up, outlook, and motivation.

Living by methodical routines is the only way to compensate for increasing forgetfulness, loss of a sense of time, the infuriating disappearance of essentials such as spectacles just when most needed, the irritability of being over-tired, and other inevitable shortcomings of ageing. It has been said that 'the peculiar value of good habits is that an individual ceases to be aware of them in a very short time and is conscious only of departure from them'. It is necessary also to be prepared to compromise if one of the habits conflicts with someone else's within the same household. The key word is method. Some lucky people are born with it, but, for most of us, to live by it is a lifelong daily struggle and, for many it is always out of reach, vanishing as they grow older. It may not be possible to escape all the worst features of mental ossification and complacency attributed to old age, but at least they can be identified and recorded by those wishing to avoid them and willing to aim at a truly 'serene sundown' in their later years.

The emphasis in advice on physical health is to avoid excess, including the extremes of hypochondriasis on one hand, and total disregard of failing health or faculties on the other. Advice is usually given on diet, exercise, sleep, and bowel habits, and on maintenance of good standards of hygiene and care of the feet. Those who need spectacles, hearing aids, or dentures are encouraged to get them without delay because, like essential operations for cataract, hernia, gynaecological repair, his replacement, or varicose veins they may be tolerated, and may prove to be more successful early rather than late in old age.

The enemies of those with cardiac insufficiency are stairs, hills and high winds. Older people who are inattentive, who have impaired postural control or defective special senses, or are liable to faints or fits must be warned about the risk of accidents and of hypothermia, and be advised to take precautions against mishaps arising from weakness and slow reaction times.

Sir Arthur Thompson (Ogilvie 1962) described health as a byproduct of activity, an amalgam of three elements: physical condition determined by good habits, activity of the mind preserved by absorbing work and stimulated by hobbies and holidays, and spiritual insight and inspiration, sought either in religious faith, or in sympathy and a sense of responsibility for others. He might have added that the effort to establish these excellent criteria in as many people as possible at every level in society is an educational ideal that should begin very early indeed.

Appendix 1

Aide-mémoire for annual re-examination of long-stay geriatric patients

1 **Brief summary of case history**
   Cause of admission, diagnosis, problems, progress, reasons for failure to leave hospital (medical, psychological, social).

2 **Update of current status**
   Routine systems' examination noting especially general condition and adenopathy, breasts, rectal examination, blood pressure, arrhythmias, CNS changes (N.B. eyes and ears).

3 **Special note of:**

Nutrition
● average
● wasted
Mobility
● walk unaided
● walk with device
● walk with help
● chairfast (transfers)
● bedfast
Pressure sores specify yes or no
● erythema
● abrasion
● ulcer
Contractures
if yes, specify
Incontinence
double/bladder only

Mental capacity
● normal
● forgetful (without constant supervision)
● confused (wandering, irresponsible, constant supervision)
● dementing (noisy, resistive, difficult)
Communication
● receptive (normal, limited, none)
● expressive
● comprehension
Behaviour
● feeding: unaided/dependent
● dressing: unaided/dependent
● personal hygiene: unaided/dependent

4 **Routine check of:**
● weight
● urine (albuminuria, glycosuria, infection)
● CBC (anaemia)
● E.S.R., Chest X-ray, EKG
● if indicated, acid and alk. phos., blood urea, electrolytes, SGOT

5 **Review of medications**

Appendix 2

ASSESSMENT FORM (GERIATRIC WARDS)

NAME				ADDRESS

AGE	SEX	M S W O	RELIGION	DIAGNOSIS (By referring physician)

SURGERY HOURS OR SUITABLE TIME TO CONTACT	DOCTOR'S NAME, ADDRESS & TELEPHONE No.

DIRECTIONS:

INFORMATION FROM DOCTOR REFERRING PATIENT. RING CONDITIONS WHICH APPLY.

Mental State	Activity	Incontinence	Contractures
Alert	Unrestricted	Urine	Legs
Slightly confused	Restricted	Faeces	Arms
Confused	Bedfast: weeks	Both	
Noisy	years	Bedsores	

NEXT OF KIN	RELATIVES	HOME CONDITIONS	
Husband/wife	Helpful	Own Home	Living alone
Son/daughter	Unco-operative	With relatives	Help from neighbours
Brother/sister	Unable to cope	Hostel	Help from relatives
Distant		Lodgings	No help
None			

PROBABLE RESULT	REQUEST FOR ADMISSION PROMPTED BY:
Home when fit	
Welfare Residential Home	
Long-stay Hospital Care	

OTHER INFORMATION

DATE	INFORMED VISIT WILL PROBABLY BE ON	SIGNED

DATE: TIME VISITED: SOCIAL WORKER: PLACE:

HOUSE and HOUSEHOLD

RELATIVES/NEIGHBOURS INTERVIEWED and ATTITUDE:

HISTORY:

MENTAL STATE and BEHAVIOUR:

PHYSICAL STATE:

DIAGNOSIS	ACTION ADVISED	SIGNED

Bibliography

ADAMS, G. F. (1974a). *Cerebrovascular disability and the ageing brain*. Churchill Livingstone, London.
—— (1974b). Eld health. *Br. med. J.* iii, 789–91.
—— (1976). Grading of recovery from strokes. *Age and Ageing* **4**, 137–41.
ADAMS, J. H. (1979). The pathology of ischaemic stroke. *Age and Ageing* **8**, Supplement, 57–66.
ADAMS, R. D. (1958). Recent advances in cerebrovascular disease. *Br. med. J.* i, 785–8.
—— (1975). The etiology of dementing diseases and special aspects of ageing. *Proceedings of the Eisenhower Medical Centre, California.*
AGATE, J. N. (1972). *The practice of geriatrics*, 2nd ed. Heinemann, London.
ALLISON, R. S. (1962). *The senile brain*. Edward Arnold, London.
—— (1964). *Mental impairment in the aged*. M. Jacobs, Philadelphia.
AMULREE, LORD (1951). *Adding life to years*. National Council of Social Service, London.
ANDERSON, SIR FERGUSON (1973). In 'Care of the dying'. *Br. med. J.*, i, 29–41.
—— (1976). *The practical management of the elderly*, 3rd ed. Blackwell, Oxford.
ANONYMOUS (a country doctor) (1964). *Facing retirement*. Allen and Unwin, London.
ASHER, R. (1947). The dangers of going to bed. *Br. med. J.* ii, 967–8.
—— (1960). Clinical sense. *Br. med. J.* i, 985–93.
BEDFORD, P. D. (1959). General medical aspects of confusional states in elderly people. *Br. med. J.* ii, 185–8.
BIANCHINE, J. R. (1976). Drug therapy of Parkinsonism. *New Engl. J. Med.* **295**, 814–18.
BLISS, M. R., MCLAREN, R., and EXTON-SMITH, A. N. (1966). Ministry of Health Bulletin, Vol. 25. H.M.S.O., London.
British Medical Journal (1977). Leading article 'The old in the cold'. i, 336.
BROCKLEHURST, J. C. (1951). *Incontinence in old people*. Livingstone, Edinburgh.
—— (1978). *Textbook of geriatric medicine and gerontology*, 2nd ed. Churchill Livingstone, Edinburgh.
BROMLEY, D. B. (1978). *The psychology of ageing*, 2nd ed. Penguin Books, Harmondsworth.
BURNET, F. M. (1970). An immunological approach to ageing. *Lancet* ii, 358–60.
BUTTERFIELD, W. H. J., KEEN, H., and WHICHELOW, M. J. (1967). Renal glucose threshold variations with age. *Br. med. J.* iv, 505–7.
CAIRD, F. I. (1979). Investigation of the elderly patient with stroke. *Age and Ageing* **8**, Supplement, 44–9.

——, and JUDGE, T. G. (1979). *The assessment of the elderly patient.* Pitman Medical, London.

——, PIRIE, A., and RAMSELL, T. G. (1969). *Diabetes and the eye.* Blackwell, Oxford.

CALNE, D. B. (1970). *Parkinsonism. Physiology, pharmacology and treatment.* Edward Arnold, London.

CLARK, A. N. G., MANKIKAR, G. D., and GRAY, I. (1975). Diogenes syndrome. A clinical study of gross neglect in old age. *Lancet* i, 366–8.

CORDAY, E., ROTHENBERG, S. F., and PUTNAM, T. J. (1953). Cerebral vascular insufficiency. *A.M.A. Archs Neurol. Psychiatry* **69**, 551–70.

CRITCHLEY, M. (1931). The neurology of old age. *Lancet* i, 1121–221.

—— (1970). *Aphasiology.* Edward Arnold, London.

DALL, J. L. (1970). Maintenance digoxin in elderly patients. *Br. med. J.* ii, 705–6.

DANON, D. and SHOCK, N. W. (1981). *Aging: A Challenge to Science and Society. Vol. 1: Biology.* Oxford University Press.

DAVISON, W. M. (1973). The hazards of drug treatment in old age, in *Textbook of geriatric medicine and gerontology* (ed. J. C. Brocklehurst), pp. 632–48. Churchill Livingstone, Edinburgh.

ECKSTEIN, D. (1976). Common complaints of the elderly. *Hosp. Pract.* April 1976.

EVERITT, A. V. (1981). Pituitary Function and Aging. In *Aging: A Challenge to Science and Society, Vol. 1 Biology* (ed. D. Danon and N. W. Shock). Oxford University Press.

EXTON-SMITH, A. N., AGATE, J. N., CROCKETT, G. S., IRVINE, R. E., and WALLIS, M. U. (1964). Accidental hypothermia in the elderly. *Br. med. J.* ii, 1255–8.

EXTON-SMITH, A. N. and OVERSTALL, P. (1979). *Guidelines in Medicine Vol. 1: Geriatrics.* MTP Press, Lancaster.

FLETCHER, C. (1980). Listening and talking to patients. *Br. med. J.* iv, 931–3; 994–6.

FOX, R. H., WOODWARD, P. M., FRY, A. J., and COLLINS, J. C. (1971). Diagnosis of accidental hypothermia of the elderly. *Lancet* i, 424–7.

GILCHRIST, A. R. (1963). The compleat physician. *Lancet* ii, 1–4.

GODBER, C. (1975). The physician and the confused elderly patient. *J. R. Coll. Physcns* **10**, 101–12.

GRANT, W. R. (1963). *Principles of rehabilitation.* E. & S. Livingstone, Edinburgh and London.

HAKIM, A. M. and MATHIESON, G. (1978). Basis of Dementia in Parkinson's disease. *Lancet* ii, 729.

HAYFLICK, L. (1965). The limited *in vitro* lifetime of human diploid cell strains. *Exp. Cell. Res.* **37**, 614–36.

—— (1974). Cytogerontology. In *Theoretical aspects of aging* (ed. M. Rockstein), pp. 83–103. Academic Press, New York.

—— (1976). The cell biology of human aging. *New Engl. J. Med.* **295**, 1302–8.

HORNYKIEWICZ, O. (1975). Parkinson's disease and its chemotherapy. *Biochem. Pharmacol.* **24**, 1064–5.

HORROBIN, D. F. (1968). *Medical physiology and biochemistry.* Edward Arnold, London.

HURWITZ, L. J. (1964). Improving mobility in severely disabled Parkinsonian patients. *Lancet* ii, 953–5.

HURWITZ, N. (1969). Predisposing factors in adverse reactions to drugs. *Br. med. J.* i, 536–9.

IRVINE, R. E., BAGNALL, M. K., and SMITH, B. J. (1968). *The older patient.* English Universities Press, London.

JARRETT, R. J. (1973). The treatment of mild, late-onset diabetes mellitus. In *Ninth Symposium on Advanced Medicine* (ed. G. Walker). Pitman Medical, London.

—— (1976). Epidemiology of diabetes. *Br. J. Hosp. Med.* **16**, 200–4.

JONES, F. A. (1972). *Richard Asher talking sense.* Pitman Medical, London.

JUDGE, T. G. (1971). The clinical importance of normal senescence. *Mod. Geriatrics* **1**, 182–7.

KAY, D. W. K., BEAMISH, P., and ROTH, M. (1964). Old age mental disorders in Newcastle upon Tyne. A study of prevalence. *Br. J. Phychiat.* **110**, 146–58.

KEELE, C. A. and NEIL, E. (1973). *Samson Wright's Applied Physiology*, 12th edn. Oxford University Press.

KENNEDY, A. (1957). Individual reactions to change as seen in senior management in industry. *Lancet* i, 261–3.

KREMER, M. (1958). Sitting, standing, and walking. *Br. med. J.* ii, 121–6.

LOWTHER, C. P., MACLEOD, R. S. M., and WILLIAMSON, J. (1970). Evaluation of early diagnostic services for the elderly. *Br. med. J.* iii, 275–7.

MACKINTOSH, J. M. (1954). The threshold of age. *Lancet* i, 991–4.

MAHLER, R. J. (1975). Differential diagnosis of impaired mental function. *Proceedings of the Eisenhower Medical Centre, California.*

MATTHEWS, W. B. (1975). *Practical neurology*, 3rd ed. Blackwell, Oxford.

MELMAN, K. L. and MORRELLI, H. F. (1978). *Clinical pharmacology*, 2nd ed. Macmillan, New York.

McKEOWN, F. (1965). *Pathology of the aged.* Butterworths, London.

NEWMAN, J. L. (1962). Old folk in wet beds. *Brit. med. J.* i, 1824–8.

OGILVIE, SIR HENEAGE (1962). *Fifty: an approach to the problems of middle age.* Max Parrish, London.

ORDY, J. M. (1981). Neurotransmitters and aging in the human brain. In *Aging: A Challenge to Science and Society Vol. 1: Biology* (ed. D. Danon and N. W. Shock). Oxford University Press.

OVERSTALL, P. (1978). *Falls in the elderly* (ed. B. Isaacs). Recent Advances in Geriatric Medicine. Churchill Livingstone, London.

PEARCE, I. and PEARCE, J. M. S. (1978). Bromocriptine in parkinsonism. *Br. med. J.* ii, 1402–4.

PEARCE, J. M. S. (1978). Aetiology and natural history of Parkinson's disease, *Br. med. J.* 2, 1664–66.

PEARSON, L. (1974). *Death and dying.* Case Western Reserve University, Cleveland and London.

PLATT, R. (1963a). Reflections on ageing and death. *Lancet* i, 1–6.

—— (1963*b*). Doctor and patient. *Lancet* ii, 1156–8.

ROCKSTEIN, M. (1974). *Theoretical aspects of aging.* Academic Press, New York.

SAUNDERS, C. (1963). The treatment of intractable pain. *Proc. R. Soc. Med.* **56**, 3, 195.

—— (1978). *The management of terminal disease.* Edward Arnold, London.

SCHEIBEL, M. E. and SCHEIBEL, A. B. (1981). Structural alterations in the aging brain. In *Aging: A Challenge to Science and Society, Vol. 1: Biology* (ed. D. Danon and N. W. Shock). Oxford University Press.

SHARP, G. L., BUTTERFIELD, W. H. J., and KEEN, H. (1964). Diabetic Survey in Bedford. *Proc. R. Soc. med.* **57**, 193–202.

SHAW, K. M., LEES, A. J., and STERN, G. M. (1980). The impact of treatment with levadopa on Parkinson's disease. *Quart. med. J.* **195**, 283–93.

SHELDON, J. H. (1948). *The social medicine of old age.* Oxford University Press, London.

—— (1950). The role of the aged in modern society. *Br. med. J.* i, 319–23.

—— (1960). On the natural history of falls in old age. *Br. med. J.* ii, 1685–90.

—— (1966). Falls in old age, in *Medicine in old age* (ed. J. N. Agate). Pitman Medical, London.

SHEPPARD, H. L. (1981). The allocation of work time over a longer life-span. In *Aging: A Challenge to Science and Society Vol. 2: Medicine and social sciences* (ed. A. J. J. Gilmore *et al.*). Oxford University Press.

SHOCK, N. W. (1962). The physiology of ageing. *Scient. Am.* **206**, 100–10.

—— (1974). Physiological theories of aging. In *Theoretical aspects of aging* (ed. M. Rockstein). Academic Press, New York.

SIMPSON, R. G. (1974). Disease patterns in the elderly. *Br. J. Hosp. Med.* **12**, 660–77.

STEVENS, D. L. and MATTHEWS, W. B. (1973). Cryptogenic drop attacks: an affliction of women. *Br. med. J.* i, 439–42.

STOKER SIR, MICHAEL (1980). New medicine and new biology. *Br. med. J.* **281**, 1678–82.

VERBOV, J. (1974). *Skin diseases in the elderly.* Heinemann, London.

WADE, O. L. (1972). Drug therapy in the elderly. *Age and Ageing* **1**, 65–73.

WALFORD, R. L. (1981). Immunoregulatory systems and aging. In *Aging: A Challenge to Science and Society. Vol. 1: Biology* (ed. D. Danon and N. W. Shock). Oxford University Press.

WALTON, SIR JOHN (1977). *Brain's diseases of the nervous system* (8th edn.). Oxford University Press.

WELFORD, A. T. (1962). On changes of performance with age. *Lancet* i, 335–58.

—— (1981). Perception, memory, and motor performance in relation to age. In *Aging: A Challenge to Science and Society. Vol. 1: Biology* (ed. D. Danon and N. W. Shock). Oxford University Press.

WILLIAMSON, J. and JOHNSON, D. B. (1980). Ageing. In *A companion to medical studies* (2nd ed.) (ed. R. Passmore and J. S. Robson). Blackwell Scientific Publications, Oxford.

WILLINGTON, F. L. (1976). *Incontinence in the elderly.* Academic Press, London.

WILSON, T. S. (1948). Urinary incontinence in the aged. *Lancet* ii, 374–7.

—— (1976). A practical approach to the treatment of incontinence of urine in the elderly, in *Incontinence in the elderly* (ed. F. L. Willington). Academic Press, London.

WRIGHT, W. B. and SIMPSON, J. H. (1967). The case for geriatrics. *Lancet* ii, 507–8.

YEATES, W. K. (1976). Normal and abnormal bladder function. In *Incontinence in the elderly* (ed. F. L. Willington). Academic Press, London.

Index

mental disorder—*continued*
  and accidental hypothermia, 71
  and assessment visits, 116–17
  and bedsores, 82
  and day hospital care, 32, 118
  and digitalis intoxication, 102
  drug-induced, 36–7, 102–3
  and incontinence, 78
metabolic bone disease, 87–90
method,
  and health in retirement, 126
micturition, physiology of, 75
milieu intérieur, 2, 9, 42, 70
mitosis,
  and cellular ageing, 2, 3, 4
morbidity, rise with age, 20–3
motivation, 26, 28
  and assessment of stroke, 46
motor impersistence in dementia, 39
motor neuron disease, 24, 52
multi-infarct dementia, 12, 24, 37, 39
multiple pathology, 23–4, 29, 84
muscle-joint sense, and walking, 49, 51
  and precision movement, 125
  and posture, 13, 49–50
mutation,
  and cell ageing, 4–5
myasthenia gravis, 53
myocardial infarction (*see* cardiac infarction)
myopathy, causes of, 53
myxoedema (and hypothyroidism), 19, 24, 27, 36, 38, 52, 53, 74, 117
  and hypothermia, 71

neglect,
  of hemiplegic limbs, 47
  social, 21, 25, 28
  and terminal illness, 91
neoplasm, 9, 36, 79 (*see also* cancer, carcinoma *and* tumour)
neuralgia,
  post-herpetic, 98, 109
  trigeminal, 98
neural peptides, 8–9, 58
neurochemistry,
  and dementia, 38
  and stroke, 41
  and parkinsonism, 57–8, 61
neuro-endocrine control,
  and ageing, 8, 9
  and homeostasis, 19
neurogenic bladder, types of, 75
neuron,
  degeneration of and ageing, 13
neurofibrillary tangles, 13, 38
neuropathy, 14
  and difficulty in walking, 53
  and falls, 55

neuropil—loss of, 8, 13
neurotransmission,
  altered by mutation, 4
  and autonomic dysfunction, 14
  and dementia, 38
  and neuro-endocrine control, 8–9
normal pressure hydrocephalus, 37

obesity, 27, 30, 74
  and antidiabetic drugs, 54
  and diabetes, 65
  and drug metabolism, 101
  and pressure sores, 81
obstructive lung (airways) disease, 16, 36
oedema,
  and blistering disorders, 110
  and gravitational eczema, 108
  and heart failure, 27
  and malnutrition, 84
oestrogen, 19, 70
olivopontocerebellar degeneration, 52, 57
on–off phenomenon and parkinsonism, 62, 63
organic brain disease, and mental disorders of old age, 35
orientation, 34
osteoarthritis, 15, 27
osteomalacia, 15, 27, 86, 87, 89–91
  diagnosis, 87
  treatment, 88–9
osteoporosis, 15, 26, 27, 87–9
  aetiology, 87
  causes of bone loss, 87–8
  and diagnosis, 88
  treatment, 88–9

Paget's disease, 15, 87, 90–1
Paget's disease of nipple, 106
pain,
  bone, in Paget's disease, 91
  control of, 97–9
  impaired sensitivity to, 13, 14, 25, 30
  mental pain, 94, 99
  metastatic bone, 98
  post-hemiplegic, 98
  in terminal illness, 93, 94
  unidentified, 36, 94, 116
pancreatitis, in hypothermia, 72
paraesthesiae, 36, 53
  and diabetes, 66, 68
  in polyarteritis nodosa, 53
  and vitamin B deficiency, 85
  and subacute combined degeneration, 51
paralysis agitans, *see* parkinsonism
paranoia, 35, 63, 116, 118
paraplegia, spastic, 51, 71, 74, 91
parkinsonism, 24, 27, 37, 39, 50, 52, 57–65, 71, 102, 112, 117, 118
  clinical picture, 58–9